Terri Salt

TOWARDS
Outstanding

A Self-Development
Reflection Workbook

Towards Outstanding
A Self-Development Reflection Workbook

© Pavilion Publishing & Media

The author has asserted her rights in accordance with the Copyright, Designs and Patents Act (1988) to be identified as the author of this work.

Published by:
Pavilion Publishing and Media Ltd
Blue Sky Offices, 25 Cecil Pashley Way
Shoreham-by-Sea, West Sussex
BN43 5FF

Tel: 01273 434 943
Email: info@pavpub.com
Web: www.pavpub.com

Published 2021

A catalogue record for this book is available from the British Library.

ISBN: 978-1-913414-73-3

Pavilion Publishing and Media is a leading publisher of books, training materials and digital content in mental health, social care and allied fields. Pavilion and its imprints offer must-have knowledge and innovative learning solutions underpinned by sound research and professional values.

Author: Terri Salt
Production editor: Mike Benge, Pavilion Publishing and Media Ltd
Cover design: Emma Dawe, Pavilion Publishing and Media Ltd
Page layout and typesetting: Emma Dawe, Pavilion Publishing and Media Ltd
Printing: Ashford Press

Contents

Part 1: Introduction

Introduction

Disclaimer

I have written this book based on far too many years' experience of health and social care and regulation. A number of my example's pre-date the establishment of the current regulator for England – the Care Quality Commission – but I hope the messages to be drawn from reflecting on them may prove useful in considering how to improve the experience of the people that you care for. Good care hasn't changed much over the years; it has evolved and become more accountable, but the underpinning foundations of compassion, kindness, team working, attention to detail and personal preferences remain as true today as ever.

This book is my work and has not been endorsed by the Commission. I rather hope that there is nothing contained within that would be at odds with the views of others who work in health or social care, or with the regulations, and that the key messages allow reflection on how well a service meets the expectations of the legislative framework, but I am not going to tell you in detail how to run your service, nor can I to give you an unearned advantage in the inspection process.

Simply reading this book isn't going to get you an improved rating. I have no influence over that process, there is a strict quality assurance and benchmarking process, whereby inspection ratings are agreed. I hope you do get improved ratings. If you are reading this book, the chances are we are on the same side and we both want people to experience high quality care. The premise of the book is that providers and staff will reflect with honesty on how they deliver care and treatment and then use those reflections to drive improvements. There are no guarantees: You and your staff have to put the effort into understanding yourselves and your own service, being honest about shortcomings and recognising the strengths so that you can build on them. The book will hopefully guide you towards an understanding of where you need to travel but it is not a free ticket. There is no easy ride to excellence. Indeed, putting the work in and seeing the fruits of your labours is part of the joy that comes with improved outcomes. It offers a way of thinking, not a replacement for thinking.

Information produced by public bodies in the UK, such as the Care Quality Commission, NHS England and the Department of Health and Social Care is included and used in accordance with the Open Government Licence v3.0.

The licencing conditions can be found at http://www.nationalarchives.gov.uk/doc/open-government-licence/version/3/

Information produced by the Care Quality Commission can be found at https://cqc.org.uk/

The context

The Towards Outstanding series of books and training materials is intended to support services in England that are registered with the Care Quality Commission to provide regulated activities. They should have applicability to all sectors, and materials can be adapted to make them more relevant to specific organisations. They are not so closely aligned to the inspection methodologies that they will become less useable as the way inspections are carried out changes – this will inevitably happen over time, but the basis of good care is timeless. The global impact of the Coronavirus pandemic has impacted on the way services are provided and the way they are regulated. There is likely to be a move towards more remote monitoring through the use of data and intelligence – which is why it is so important to have clear evidence of what you are doing well and to share this through engagement with the regulator.

The book series does focus on the legislative framework for England, but with very little work it can be adapted to be relevant in other countries that embrace health and social care regulation as a force for bringing about improvements, particularly where ratings are given.

The Welsh regulations for providers of adult social care, for example, have significant overlap and include many of the same requirements as the regulations that providers of adult social care in England must adhere to. The Regulation and Inspection of Social Care (Wales) Act (2016) makes many similar requirements to the Health and Social Care Act (2008) (Regulated Activities) Regulations 2014.

Scotland's Health and Social Care Standards are worded differently but impose very similar requirements on providers. The Regulation and Quality Improvement Authority (RQIA) operates in Northern Ireland and while its standards are perhaps more explicit, they set the same requirements. The framework for the Health Information and Quality Authority for Ireland has more in common with the English framework than is different. While Canada has different guidance and standards for each province, the content is remarkably similar.

My experience and the case studies in the main text are predominantly from England. The messages are international and have relevance to most countries where health and social care is delivered with similar national or provincial standards. The list of English-speaking countries with aligned regulation frameworks is long and includes, but is not limited to (in no particular order):

- Canada
- Ireland
- Scotland
- Wales
- Northern Ireland
- Bahamas
- Malta and Gozo
- United Arab Emirates
- Mauritius
- South Africa
- Singapore
- Hong Kong
- Jamaica
- Australia
- USA
- India

Many non-English speaking countries also have aligned regulation of health and social care settings too, particularly across Europe.

Good care is good care regardless of where it is provided. There is a commonality of understanding among health and social care professionals the world over about what excellence looks like. Achieving it can be a little harder.

Excellence in health and social care has changed very little since I started training; it has always been about providing personalised care that meets the needs and preferences of individuals. The legal framework has changed, the level of accountability has changed, the way services are regulated has changed a little (but not as much as might be imagined) and the expectations of society have changed, but if one reads the works of long ago – Florence Nightingale wrote, "The symptoms or the sufferings generally considered to be inevitable and incident to the disease are very often not symptoms of the disease at all, but of something quite different—of the want of fresh air, or of light, or of warmth, or of quiet, or of cleanliness, or of punctuality and care in the administration of diet, of each or of all of these." If slightly more modern words were used, the statement could easily have been written by any Director of Nursing of an acute or mental health trust or any care home manager today.

From a medical perspective, Hippocrates himself said, "It's far more important to know what person the disease has than what disease the person has." The modern version of the Hippocratic oath says, "I will remember that I do not treat a fever chart, a cancerous growth, but a sick human being, whose illness may affect the person's family and economic stability. My responsibility includes these related problems, if I am to care adequately for the sick."

The basic underpinning tenets of outstanding care really have changed very little. We just need to remember them and that can be challenging in our fast-paced and ever-changing world.

Why reflect?

"By three methods we may learn wisdom: First, by reflection, which is noblest; Second, by imitation, which is easiest; and third by experience which is bitterest."
Confucius

"Self-reflection entails asking yourself questions about your values, assessing your strengths and failures, thinking about your perceptions and interactions with others, and imagining where you want to take your life in the future."
Robert L. Rosen

Reflective practice helps people think about their experiences and actions in order to be better at what we do. It uses a process of looking at our own experiences and how our behaviour and actions impact on situations. It allows for continuous learning.

Reflective practice helps us to see and accept that we look at current experiences through individual lenses of prior experiences. It helps us see that the way we think and behave, the assumptions we make, are what create our organisational culture and norms. It helps us understand why we hold certain beliefs and why we act in certain ways. Learning can only really embed if we challenge our own perceptions and beliefs and are honest with ourselves about what we do well and where we could improve. Understanding how our behaviour and attitudes affect others can help improve communications and outcomes in all areas of our lives. Those who have experience of coaching or of being coached will see that it is almost a way of coaching ourselves towards improvement.

Recognising our individual and team practice, what we do well and building on that is a joyful experience. It is good to recognise good practice and allow ourselves to take pleasure in what we do well.

It is also important that we look at where we could make improvements, where we have made mistakes (and why). Thinking about where something went wrong – be it a conversation, a prescription, an omission of care or a Never Event – and understanding our part in that mistake, can help us prevent the same thing happening again.

For that to be truly effective we cannot rely on a change of policy (although that might be necessary); we must assume responsibility for our own actions. If a new policy is introduced, we must take responsibility for reading and understanding it, and we must make sure we follow it, but reflective practice goes further. We must think about our contribution to a mistake or omission of care and at least be honest with ourselves. Were we distracted by a call from our childminder and forgot that Mr Smith had asked for some analgesia? Did we go to examine Mrs Jones' leg because the night staff said it was painful and swollen, but on finding she wasn't there started doing discharge letters and only remember about Mrs Jones when she collapsed with chest pain and breathing difficulties?

Reflective practice can help us understand our own intentions, values and visions and support us to work in a challenging field where our ethics and morals may be tested, where power relations may be decidedly unequal, and where we may be working in emotionally and physically demanding environments. This has never been truer than at the present time (April, 2020) when we are amid a global pandemic that requires a Herculean response from health and social care staff. Hopefully, as we move forward, there will be time to reflect and think about the impact on our staff, our patients and their families. Reflection will not change what has happened this time, but will help us to build resilience and to be better prepared in the event of a future pandemic or other crisis. That reflection might also help staff who are feeling despair to recognise how incredibly well they have coped, and how many lives they have saved. Hopefully, they will see that the strategies they used to cope may be transferred to other times and situations.

Many of us keep coming back to questions about how we can make a difference. It is, after all, the reason most people entered health and social care. The truth is that each and every one of us can make a difference. We might not be a CEO; we might sometimes feel insignificant in large and complex organisations, but how you approach your work makes a huge difference to individuals using services. The woman in labour, the person who has vomited, the person who has fallen and cut their forehead, is not going to remember an executive director. They will remember the staff who were kind, who were compassionate and who made them feel safe.

Practicing reflection can help us answer these questions and others throughout our lives and careers.

We might feel powerless and feel it is always outside our control when things are not right, but that is rarely the case. We have far more influence than we think – albeit sometimes within a small sphere of influence.

Imagine you are a frail, elderly, Sudanese woman who has fallen and has been brought into the emergency department by ambulance, soaked in urine because you had lain on the floor for a long time, in pain and distress. Your daughter, who normally brings your shopping, helps you shower and fits your hearing aids, is on holiday for a week. Your glasses were broken in the fall. Don't just read it, really imagine it… What might you be feeling? How might the situation impact on your behaviour? What if you had difficulty understanding English? What would you be wanting to happen? How would you want to be cared for?

Now think about your approach and how this could impact on the experience and possibly the outcomes for that particular patient. You can easily change it to other care settings if you can't imagine a hospital emergency department. Try thinking about the same woman being discharged from hospital to your care home or referred to your fall assessment service. Imagine she is trying to get an appointment at your GP practice. What would make you go home thinking you had really helped her have a favourable impression of your service? What could you do that would result in her telling her daughter about how kind you were?

Reflective practice can also be a particularly powerful tool for organisational learning and for monitoring service quality. It can be used to evaluate the impact of training or to ensure staff understand and are following good practice. It's not simply enough to complete training; it's learning from the training that is important, surely?

Within the Care Quality Commission inspection framework under the 'Safe' key question there is quite a strong emphasis on the reporting, investigation and learning from incidents. That is about organisational reflection and making changes to reduce the risk of recurrence. Across all directorates and types of services, there is a focus on recognition, reporting, investigation and learning from incidents. Those services which provide the very best care and treatment are those services that are open to staff raising concerns, identifying mistakes or spotting risks, reporting these without fear of censure and where they feel something will be done about it. They are the organisations which encourage staff and teams to reflect, to be honest and comprehensive about the possible causes of mistakes – rather than defensive – and where they share the learning widely rather than write up a superficial report then hide it away in a filing cabinet.

There cannot be effective organisational reflection without individual and team reflection. It is not about apportioning blame or scapegoating – or at least it should not be. Any organisation where staff feel they will not be listened to is a long way from being outstanding.

CQC key lines of enquiry
Adult Social Care

What are the arrangements for reviewing and investigating safety and safeguarding incidents and events when things go wrong? Are all relevant staff, services, partner organisations and people who use services involved in reviews and investigations?

How are lessons learned and themes identified, and is action taken as a result of reviews and investigations when things go wrong?

CQC key lines of enquiry
Hospitals

What are the arrangements for reviewing and investigating safety and safeguarding incidents and events when things go wrong? Are all relevant staff, services, partner organisations and people who use services involved in reviews and investigations?

How are lessons learned and themes identified, and is action taken as a result of investigations when things go wrong?

How well is the learning from lessons shared to make sure that action is taken to improve safety? Do staff participate in and learn from reviews and investigations by other services and organisations?

Reflection can also be used for addressing issues of conflict, resistance and misuse of power in relationships, which are often present as barriers to individual and organisational development, but which are seldom dealt with directly. The reflection is the tool for helping people understand the impact of their behaviour and action – it has to come from the people involved and cannot be imposed or one-sided. It can, and should be, a part of other processes – supervision, performance management, coaching, mentoring, revalidation, mediation, induction, leadership development, training and quality monitoring. While leaders, mentors, coaches and managers cannot reflect on someone else's behalf, they can ask the questions and encourage the member of staff to reflect.

Keeping a reflective journal is a way to reflect through documenting ideas, feelings, observations and visions. This journal is a first step into the world of reflection and is not intended to be a finite resource. It is simply something to focus and lead you into a process of reflection, to help understand yourself, your work or your team better.

Used properly and honestly, it should help you become increasingly self-aware and honest with yourself. Over time, I hope you develop your own ways of reflecting, which might well be a page-a-day diary where you make notes about your day and go back with a different coloured pen to reflect on what you did or felt after the moment had passed and any immediate feelings had dissipated. It could be a ring binder or wallet file in which you store feedback and reflect on that. It might be a computer file with your immediate thoughts and reflections.

This journal is personal. You can't get it wrong. It is what you think and feel. It isn't something to be marked as correct or otherwise. There is no score chart. There is no right answer. You simply need to be honest with yourself about your thoughts and feelings, and then open to looking at things from a different perspective, open to challenge from yourself and others who may hold a different viewpoint. Fixed mindsets – "We tried that before and it doesn't work" or "We haven't got time for that" – are significant barriers to overcome and allow changes to be introduced. Very rarely are things 'cut and dried', especially in the complex and ever-changing world of health and social care.

People are entitled to different views and we need to become comfortable with difference if we want to understand ourselves and others. How the mother of three young children perceives a trumpet being played loudly and not very well from the neighbouring house at 9pm is likely to be at variance with the view of the recently retired, enthusiastic beginner who she lives next door to. Reflection helps us understand our reactions and how others might be feeling. That can make life nicer for us all.

The journal is not intended to be handed over to anyone else without you requesting they look at it. It might be that your organisation wants to run a series of reflective learning days and to use the journal as a supporting tool, but the actual journal remains private. If you know it is going to be seen by trainers, peers or managers you might not be quite so frank; the risk is you write what you think people want to read, rather than your reality.

Sharing and reflecting together is good. It brings balance and challenge. Individual challenge and reflection can help us avoid making the same mistakes twice: I remember making a decision to start the journey to my children's nursery school 15 minutes earlier after I reflected on a very embarrassing lecture about speeding from a police officer on the school driveway, in full view of all the other parents dropping off children.

Shared reflection really is better: when I talked to my husband about it (OK, in truth, when my eldest daughter talked to her father about it), we decided to ensure the morning nursery drop off was less of a rush. I left 15 minutes earlier, made possible by ensuring I had put the uniform out the previous evening and by my husband defrosting and warming the car on his way out to work. I was then less rushed and calmer, which meant I was nicer to the children, so they had fewer 'meltdowns' as they were pushed out of the door. Life became more pleasant for us all and I avoided any further embarrassing lectures.

I was pushed into sharing by a daughter who thought it was the funniest thing ever to see mummy squirming. Although I might not have shared had I not been pushed, it meant we could work together on a solution and that we both took ownership of a joint responsibility.

The sharing should take place in a setting that feels comfortable and where there are clear rules around listening, accepting difference, refraining from personal insults or attack and not using things heard in the group to belittle others. Clearly, if there are safeguarding issues or entirely inappropriate language or behaviours used, these need addressing, but education has always been the most powerful tool for bringing about changes. Telling someone not to make an overtly ageist comment is less likely to bring about a change of attitude than helping them see that there is no such thing as 'the elderly', but that there are many very different elderly people. Being reminded that the Queen rides her horse at 95 years of age, may remind us that not everyone over 70 years of age needs a plastic beaker.

Keeping a reflective journal can help you to:

■ focus your thoughts and develop your ideas about what good practice looks like
■ develop your voice and gain confidence at sharing your ideas and concerns
■ experiment with ideas and ask questions; use it as a sounding board
■ organise your thinking through exploring complex issues
■ develop your skills in analysing and using information
■ reflect upon experiences and understand the processes behind them
■ express your feelings and emotional responses in an acceptable way
■ become aware of your actions and strategies and how these impact upon care.

When keeping a reflective journal:

■ write for yourself; this is your reflection
■ be informal, using language you are comfortable with; say what you really think
■ write in your own first language; it is for you to understand not for others
■ be relaxed and comfortable; it's sometimes better not to record immediately, perhaps if you are angry or upset
■ use diagrams and drawings to remind yourself of the details

- reflect not just on events, but on processes and relationships
- ask questions and challenge assumptions of yourself and others
- connect personal and professional experiences to concepts and theories, although not necessarily at the early stages of learning to reflect; it's the reflection that is important.

The professional consensus is that reflection is a positive thing that supports individual, group and organisational learning.

The Health and Care Professionals Council issued a statement in June 2019, jointly with eight other professional regulatory bodies including the General Dental Council, the General Medical Council, the Nursing and Midwifery Council, the General Optical Council, the General Pharmaceutical Council, the General Osteopathic Council, the Health and Care Professionals Council, the General Chiropractic Council and the Pharmaceutical Council for Northern Ireland. I have set it out below:

> *"This joint statement sets out our common expectations for health and care professionals to be reflective practitioners, engaging meaningfully in reflection and the benefits it brings.*
>
> *Being a reflective practitioner benefits people using health and care services by:*
>
> - *Supporting individual professionals in multi-disciplinary teamwork.*
> - *Fostering improvements in practice and services.*
> - *Assuring the public that health and care professionals are continuously learning and seeking to improve.*
>
> *As well as expecting the people we regulate to be reflective practitioners, we also have a duty to consider our own actions, and their effect. We are committed to improving how we provide assurance and protection to the public. We do this continuously in our work, through evaluation, to reflect and make changes in what we do and how we work. This statement reflects the principles set out in each regulator's individual code of practice, professional standards or guidance on reflective practice.*
>
> *Reflective practice allows an individual to continually improve the quality of care they provide and gives multi-disciplinary teams the opportunity to reflect and discuss openly and honestly.*

Reflection is the thought process where individuals consider their experiences to gain insights about their whole practice. Reflection supports individuals to continually improve the way they work or the quality of care they give to people. It is a familiar, continuous and routine part of the work of health and care professionals.

Opportunities for multi-professional teams to reflect and discuss openly and honestly what has happened when things go wrong should be encouraged. These valuable reflective experiences help to build resilience, improve well-being and deepen professional commitment."

The statement affirms that reflection plays an important role in healthcare, and brings benefits to service users by:

- fostering improvements in practices and services
- assuring the public that health and care professionals are continuously learning and seeking to improve.

The statement reinforces that reflection is a key element of development and educational requirements and, in some professions, for revalidation as well.

It also makes clear that service user confidentiality is vital, and that registrants will never be asked to provide their personal reflective notes to investigate a concern about them.

The statement makes clear that teams should be encouraged to make time for reflection, as a way of aiding development, improving well-being and deepening professional commitment. There is also a professional requirement for health and social care practitioners to use reflection as a tool for improving their own practice.

The Nursing and Midwifery Council (NMC) requires that nurses and midwives use feedback as an opportunity for reflection and learning, to improve practice. The NMC revalidation process requires that registrants provide examples of how they have achieved this.

The GMC has produced guidance called *The Reflective Practitioner: Guidance for doctors and medical students*, which makes clear the expectation that doctors use reflection throughout their careers.

Reflecting on experiences and practice is vital to personal well-being and development, and to improving the quality of patient care. Experiences, both good and bad, have learning potential for the individuals involved and for the wider system.

Finally, reflecting is good for mental well-being and building resilience, with the caveat that it needs to be done with a positive attitude. It isn't helpful to look back at every interaction, every action, and to dissect them forensically or to use mistakes to beat yourself or others up. It's never about looking to blame yourself nor to dump responsibility entirely onto others and dismiss the very notion you might have helped avoid errors or poor outcomes by changing the way you behaved or reacted.

It is about developing self-awareness and knowing your strengths, so that you can build on them and possibly shine a light for others to see what best practice looks like.

Allowing yourself to be pleased with how you did something challenging or how well you maintained a calmness in the face of difficulties is a good thing. Too often we focus on small failings instead of the myriad of good things we do.

Reflection can be hugely enjoyable and a real boost to morale. It builds integrity and a culture where people can ask for help or admit errors safely, at a stage where things can be put right. It builds the confidence of individuals and the team. It gives a shared understanding and shared learning, which in turn improves professional and personal relationships.

There are no negatives to learning – and reflection, where we develop an ability to question ourselves, is a giant leap towards becoming our very best.

Using this journal

How you use this journal is entirely up to you and your employer (if they have provided it for your learning). It has value as a stand-alone log of your own reflection but is primarily intended as a supporting tool alongside a course of shared reflective learning. Sharing reflections and learning from each other is the most effective way to reshape our thinking and to modify our approach. It offers independent challenge and a wider perspective.

This journal isn't complicated. Our time is often our most precious resource and hopefully this journal, when used alongside the training pack that forms part of the *Towards Outstanding* book series, will give participants thinking and reflection time before each learning session. The learning is likely to be richer if participants have had an opportunity to think through issues before coming together. Trying to think of examples or consider your own viewpoint when 'put on the spot' is never easy. Far better we think of examples and order our thoughts and feelings ahead of the discussion.

What this journal isn't is a source of answers – they must come from within yourself and your team to be any use in driving improvements. Simply being told the best way to do something isn't terribly effective – the driver has to be an internal personal, or shared, commitment to understanding ourselves and our core values and a willingness to reconsider from a differing perspective. Thinking we always know best because we've done something for a long time, isn't the way to excellence.

The journal is broken down into separate sections aligned to the series text. It broadly aligns to the CQC inspection framework and covers many areas that an inspection covers. It focuses on the five domains of Safe, Effective, Caring, Responsive and Well-led, but won't cover all the key lines of enquiry. Once you embed the idea of reflection, it is very easy to transfer to other topics. It's even useful in your private life and can be a useful tool if you find yourself in a battle of wills with a toddler or nagging a teenager to get up earlier.

The course (or this journal) is not something to rush at and complete quickly. A ticked register of attendance at the end of ten weeks is not a mark of success. If it is to work and move you towards better practice, better experiences for people using your service and better staff engagement, then it cannot simply be a task to mark off.

You will know that you are becoming more reflective when you start asking yourself questions and having 'random thoughts' at odd times. You might be peeling potatoes when you suddenly have a lightbulb moment and think:

> *"If only I'd parked more carefully at work, I wouldn't have prevented a relative from opening their car door and going home. If they hadn't then waited ten minutes in the rain for the door to be answered, they might not have started shouting at me. Had I listened and apologised; I might not feel so bad. Instead, I was rude to them because I was embarrassed and now they've made a formal complaint".*

As a course leader or manager, you know you are getting there when a member of staff arrives and says, "I was thinking… or I've had a thought…".

Thinking and reflection take time. That doesn't necessarily mean time out of work or time sat at a desk. I do my best thinking in all sorts of strange places and at odd times. Often it is when we are walking our Dalmatian. He runs off into the sea at West Wittering, as I watch a flock of geese flying in formation. That sets me off thinking about leadership and how I am with my team and whether I could provide better support, in some way. I can then spend an hour walking around the very beautiful East Head, while at the same time planning a team meeting or thinking about how to offer development opportunities.

The opportunities for reflection are endless and can be on a bus, in bed, in the bath, while running or when flying to Dubai. All sorts of things can be triggers. That is not to say that you should never switch off or that work should always be at the forefront of your thoughts. It's simply to say you don't need special time. Any relatively calm time will do – and sometimes you can't help when it is.

If you are doing this alone or as part of a group learning session, you can choose a few questions to reflect on or look at them all. It can even be useful to look back, after a period of time, and think about whether your attitude has changed and why that might be.

Undoubtedly, the Coronavirus pandemic will alter the way individuals and organisations react and behave moving forward. While it brings huge worries and anxieties, there are opportunities for us all in amidst the horrific news stories. There will be lots of reflection and thinking, probably public enquiries too. If it means our infection prevention and control measures remain improved, that is a good thing and might reduce the number of avoidable sepsis deaths. If it results in less environmental damage because people don't want to travel internationally as much, that is also probably a good thing. Out of mistakes, problems, sadness and anger can come buds of new practice that grow and become established; they can improve things for individuals and the wider world. I'm learning a bit about gardening with the hope of producing my own raspberries, potatoes and celeriac (a bit niche, but I love the stuff). I've also rediscovered my sewing machine and have revisited my limited talents with an intent to improve. Several of my team have been gifted extremely tasteful, bespoke masks. At the end of the journal I have included a blank template that allows you to plan out how to bring about changes in your area or organisation. It gives several simple methodologies that are underpinned by a couple of recognised models of change.

Hopefully, by the time you reach the end of the journal you will have found a thirst for reflection as a tool for learning, organisational development and continuous improvement.

First impressions

"A good first impression can work wonders."
JK Rowling

Research shows that:

For individuals:

- First impressions last for months.
- First impressions impact personal judgments even in the presence of contradictory evidence about the individual.
- Studies by Princeton psychologists Janine Willis and Alexander Todorov reveal that it takes only a tenth of a second for someone to form a first impression of a stranger simply from their face.

For organisations:

If the first impression is not a positive one, then you have to work hard to overcome that initial perception. The message you are giving out is either 'We don't care what people think' or 'We think we're better than you think we are'.

You then need to spend time, effort and even money persuading the audience to see you in a better light. Unfortunately, you often do not get that chance. People quickly pass judgment on you and are likely to move on without learning what you really offer.

I know I chose my current GP practice based on reputation and first impressions. It was the reception staff that sold it to me. Luckily, that reputation holds true and the first impressions given by warm, smiling, helpful reception staff was indicative of a very good practice.

If an organisation does not project a positive first impression, the persisting view of the service will remain tainted for a considerable time. The subsequent interactions may be compromised because of the impact the first impression had.

Reflections

What impression do you want to give about yourself? What do you want people to think about you when they first meet you?

In what way does the way you present yourself support the impression you want to give?

Can you think of a time that you were perceived differently from how you wanted and why this might have been?

Does the way you want to be perceived when you meet someone differ from the first impression your organisation wants to make? Are you different at work in any way? Why?

Can you think of a time when someone else has made a bad first impression on you? Why do you think that was? How did you respond? Did you ever change that impression?

What are the implications for you, in your role at work, if you create a bad first impression?

Can you remember back to your interview? What impression did the organisation make on you and why? How did you come away feeling? What was good about it and what was less good?

If you were appointing a new member of staff, what might you have done differently?

Now think about where you work currently. What impression do you think your organisation wants to give to people using the service? Who does it want to appeal to? What would it say the preferred image was?

What impression do you think people actually have when they arrive at your work for the first time? How does this differ from the impression the organisation wants to give? Try and imagine, using several of your senses – what people might see, hear or smell? What might make them have a positive reaction? What negative feelings, if any, might people have when they first arrive?

How could the first impression for people visiting the first time be improved?

How could these improvements be achieved? Think about what your organisation or team could do, and also how you could influence this.

Now back to you: could you do anything to ensure that, on first meeting, people see you as you want to be perceived? Think about your appearance, your grooming, messages from badges or other accessories, your expression and body language, the initial interactions.

_____

_____

_____

_____

_____

How could you understand what first impression people have of you, your team or organisation?

_____

_____

_____

_____

_____

Equality and Diversity

"I have the audacity to believe that peoples everywhere can have three meals a day for their bodies, education and culture for their minds, and dignity, equality, and freedom for their spirits."

Martin Luther King, Jr

The Care Quality Commission asks its own staff, "Why do we need to consider equality and human rights in regulatory work?" That is a question everyone working in health and social care needs to ask themselves too.

The Commission gives the reasons as:

"To fulfil our purpose, we want all people using services to receive safe, effective, high quality care. There is also increasing evidence of the link between workforce equality and good quality care. This is why looking at equality for people who use services and for staff in our regulatory work is important. Equality for people using services is included in our regulations – and equality for people using services and for staff is covered in our assessment frameworks.

"The human rights principles of fairness, respect, equality, dignity and autonomy are also fundamental to good care. Many of the most serious failings in care services have been human rights breaches. Human rights principles are built into our regulations and assessment frameworks. Having a shared understanding of what these principles mean in practice, building on human rights law – and then acting to protect and promote these rights is necessary for us as a regulator. This is why human rights are important."

The five principles underpin all international human rights agreements, incorporating articles used in the Human Rights Act (1998) and are closely aligned with the Equality Act (2010). The Commission added two additional principles to the five internationally agreed principles; the human rights article of right to life, because it is so fundamental, and a principle of staff rights and empowerment, based on research that links staff empowerment to the quality of care they deliver.

Do you think there is a link between workforce equality and good care? What does this mean to you? Is your organisation equal for all staff?

_____

_____

_____

_____

_____

The Equality Act (2010) brings together numerous pieces of legislation into a single Act. The Act gives a legal framework to protect the rights of individuals and advance equality of opportunity for all.

Inequality in Health and Social Care in the UK

The Kings Fund tells us that health inequalities are avoidable, unfair and systematic differences in health between different groups of people.

Health inequalities are about differences in the people's health outcomes. The term is also used to refer to differences in the care that people receive and the opportunities that they have to lead healthy lives.

Health inequalities can mean differences in:

- *overall life expectancy and how likely people are to be affected by chronic illness*
- *access to care, such as availability of treatments and whether people can use them or have access to a GP*
- *quality and experience of care*
- *behavioural risks to health such as alcohol or drug use or smoking*
- *wider factors that affect health such as housing, employment or clean air.*

A clear example of a health inequality is around life expectancy. Men living in the least deprived areas can expect to live 9.4 years longer than men in the most deprived areas.

The Kings Fund says that the gap in healthy life expectancy at birth is stark. In 2015–17, people in the least deprived areas could expect to live roughly 19 more years in good health than those in the most deprived areas. People in the most deprived areas spend around a third of their lives in poor health, twice the proportion spent by those in the least deprived areas.

Why do you think there is significant difference between men from Blackpool (where the life expectancy is around 74.2 years) and Hart, in Hampshire, where the average life expectancy for men is 83.4 years? What factors might influence this? How does it make you feel? What could be done to reduce the gap? Is it even something you need to think about?

_____

_____

_____

_____

_____

What does equality mean for you personally, and in your work role? How are you affected? Do you see difference? Are you comfortable with difference? Do you think everyone is treated the same? Should everyone be treated the same?

_____

_____

_____

_____

_____

The British Social Attitudes Survey 2010 showed that 36% of people in the UK reported thinking sexual relations between two adults of the same sex was 'always or mostly' wrong. This increases to 50% of people who identify as religious.

The Office for National Statistics report, *Sexual orientation, UK: 2018* showed there were an estimated 1.2 million people aged 16 years and over identifying as Lesbian, Gay or Bisexual. That is 2.2% of the population.

What do you think? Does this impact on your work at all? Do you feel differently in different situations – in your personal life, what you think of colleagues, how you provide care and treatment, how you are treated? Does it change for people you know personally?

How might homophobia present in health and social care settings? Is it only relevant to sexual health or mental health services? What might the impact be? How can you help address that?

_____

_____

_____

_____

_____

_____

The same survey showed that 52% of people feared that the UK is deeply divided along religious lines. The majority were particularly concerned about Islam, compared to other faiths.

In 2018, data from the Annual Population Survey at the Great Britain level showed there were 3,372,966 people who identified as Muslim compared to an overall population of 65,288,422. By my calculations, that is marginally over 5% who class themselves as Muslim compared with 51% of the population who consider themselves to be Christian and 34% who say they have no religion.

Do those figures surprise you? If so, why?

_____

_____

_____

_____

_____

We regularly hear reports of horrific treatment that some people are subject to. In March 2019, *The Guardian* newspaper reported that the number of anti-Muslim hate crimes reported across Britain increased by 593% in the week after a white supremacist killed worshippers at two New Zealand mosques.

In 2017, a man set his dog on two Muslims during a 'campaign of racism'. His crossbreed bull terrier bit a man and left a woman traumatised. During one of the attacks, the 32-year-old shouted: "You bite her, bite her. They kill people. So, go on, bite a Muslim."

Also, in 2017, a 58-year-old Muslim man was stabbed as he arrived at the Islamic Cultural Centre on Grove Lane. Greater Manchester Police confirmed the incident is being treated as a hate crime, and that two men had been arrested in connection with the attack. The Muslim man had treated victims of the Manchester Arena bombing. After he was out of the hospital, he said that he had forgiven his attackers and that they were "not representative of what this country stands for".

How do these reports make you feel? Do they challenge your ideas and perceptions at all? Is stereotyping always a bad thing? A stereotype is a fixed general image or set of characteristics that a lot of people believe represent a particular type of person. Are there stereotypes that hold true?

Do you believe any of the following?

- *Signing isn't a language, it's English in actions.*
- *Welsh men have good singing voices.*
- *Asians are better at science and maths than Europeans.*
- *Women are more emotionally intelligent.*

Now think about whether you make assumptions about what people like or what they need and how this impacts on your approach to them. Can you think of any time when the care or treatment you provided was affected by an assumption or stereotype? Might you speak louder to old people automatically? Do you always formally assess the capacity of patients over 70 years of age admitted for elective surgery? (Which is contrary to the principles of the Mental Capacity Act (2005) – but that's another area altogether).

If a pregnant woman talks about her partner, do you assume it is a man? Do you not offer a Muslim man a sherry when the drinks trolley comes around before lunch? Do you assume a Catholic woman won't want a termination or contraception?

Your thoughts:

_____

_____

_____

_____

_____

_____

It would be rare in health or social care to work exclusively with white British colleagues. As of March 2019, 20% of the more than 1.2 million staff employed by the health service were BAME, compared with 14% of the general population of England and Wales. Among doctors, the proportion of non-British NHS staff is higher with 26% coming from overseas.

While around 84% of the adult social care workforce are British, they are not necessarily, of course, white British. There are 16% of the adult social care workforce who are not British nationals.

Can you think of the benefits staff who are foreign nationals bring to your service and the health and social care sector more widely? Think about it from an individual and a group perspective.

_____

_____

_____

_____

_____

_____

If you needed to move across a continent or the world to live in another country, what do you think would help you feel more welcome, more accepted and more 'at home'?

If you have done this, and are supporting a health or social care service as a foreign national worker, what would have made your early life in the UK easier?

Is there anything you could do (or already do) that helps include staff who come from different backgrounds to feel welcomed and accepted? Think personally and from an organisational or community perspective. Little things matter! What are the barriers that stop this happening?

In 2016, the Care Quality Commission published a report showing that certain groups in society experienced poorer quality care at the end of life because providers do not always understand or fully consider their specific needs. Subsequently, the government said that everyone should be able to access high-quality and personalised end of life care built around their individual needs and preferences. There are only a few regulated services where end of life care is not a part of their work; dying is everybody's business and there is only one opportunity to get it right. In the context of good end of life care, meeting individual needs and preferences are paramount.

Can you think about what might be important to you in your last year of life?

_____

_____

_____

Do you think these are the same as everyone else wants? If not, how might it vary from person to person?

_____

_____

_____

_____

_____

Which protected characteristics should be considered and how might they change care delivery? In what way do things like sexuality or marriage status matter when you are coming towards the end of your life?

_____

_____

_____

_____

_____

Now think about the care and treatment you provide.

End of life care might be a rare occurrence (maybe in an independent hospital), it might be you only deal with one specific aspect of care of people with a terminal illness or their families (a travel clinic offering advice for a bucket list trip, perhaps) or it might be part of your 'everyday'. How you approach it will vary but the process of thinking about how it could be more personal, more individual, how you could improve care at the end of life remains pertinent.

What do you do well and what could you do to make it better? If you had a magic wand, what might you change?

_____

_____

_____

_____

_____

Do you consider a person's, or their family's, spiritual needs? Are you comfortable talking about things like religious wishes? Would you ask a chaplain to come to your emergency department, to visit your care home, to come with you to a traveller's site? Does it make a difference if you have a faith? Is spiritual care less important than physical care?

_____

_____

_____

_____

_____

If you aren't comfortable talking about the impact of faith and spiritual care, how could you ensure that the person had their spiritual needs met? Or isn't it important? What if they have dementia or a learning disability; are they able to have a faith?

_____

_____

_____

_____

_____

Honesty and integrity

First question: what does honesty and integrity mean to you, personally and professionally? Can they be set at two different levels? Are you honest at work because you are required to be but not in your private life? Are small untruths ever justified? How comfortable are you standing up and making sure you do the right thing? What about if others disagree or your organisation isn't receptive?

Have you ever spoken up and not been listened to or felt pressure not to speak out about a concern? Have you ever felt you were being asked to be less than honest? What is the right way to raise concerns? Is it ever justified to go to the press or use social media to voice a concern about your work?

Would you feel comfortable raising a general concern about your organisation (such as not having heating on during a very cold spell)? How would you feel about raising a concern about another member of staff? Would it be different if it were a senior member of staff or your manager? How might you feel if it was someone you worked closely with?

What do you think the possible impact and risks of the following situations are and what might be a better way to have acted? Would you do anything?

1. You know your colleague has booked flights for the day before their annual leave starts. On the day they phone in sick and say they have been sick all night.

2. It's been a really busy nightshift and you know things have been missed. When you do a final check before the day staff arrive, you see that a colleague has filled in all the fluid balance charts for their patient for times when they were on their break. What is the risk around this?

3. The shift leader takes a call from the mother of a young person with learning disabilities, who is worried about their mood. The staff member says the service user has been out to their work placement all day and is a just a bit tired. You know this isn't true and that they refused to go and have spent all day in their room. What are the risks around this?

4. You become aware that data submitted to the commissioners is very inaccurate.

Part 2:
Is it safe?

Brilliant basics

"Count the Pennies and the Pounds will look after themselves."
My granny and many others

"Get the basics right first, then add those magic touches."
Linda Moir

"I try to do the right thing at the right time. They may just be little things, but usually they make the difference between winning and losing."
Kareem Abdul-Jabbar

Getting the basics right is essential before you even begin to look towards being outstanding. It is no good being an internationally renowned hospital and research centre, with fantastic outcomes for the 1 in 50,000 people who suffer from hereditary angioedema in the UK, if Great Aunt Maud is left in pain, lying in soiled bedding with her supper out of reach.

The quote from Linda Moir, above, is about the organisational philosophy when she was the cabin crew director at Virgin Atlantic. She has said "Basics are the bottom of what customers expect."

Her stance is that only once a business has the basics right can the 'magic touches' be added to make the service memorable and go beyond the basic expectations. I think most people would accept that the prospect of a Virgin Atlantic flight creates a different set of expectations and perceptions to a no-frills carrier.

I like the lovely Blue-Sky cocktail that Finn Air serve before take-off; I mention it frequently to others. I wouldn't comment on how delicious my drink was if my flights had been marred by dirty lavatories or rude staff.

If you want to be a beacon of excellence, you need to ensure the basics are right before looking skyward to a ratings grid of turquoise. That is not to suggest you should set yourself low aspirations, but rather that you need to build excellence on strong foundations. That is as true for individuals as it is for teams, or for an entire organisation.

An individual working against a culture of least effort and an attitude of 'that will do' or 'this is the way we do things', will need to be firm in their ambition to be the best. It helps to remember what is important and that is always going to be in the best interests of people using services. Giving good care and treatment feels much, much nicer than providing sub-optimal care.

Getting the basics right has huge advantages for organisations. It impacts on internal and external relationships, finances, recruitment, reputation and workforce culture. A clear, shared vision where the focus remains on the people using services will always outperform a target driven or finance driven culture – and it is more cost effective as a bonus.

The basics of good care are mainly what the 'Safe' domain of an inspection are all about. If you aren't offering safe care, then you simply cannot be outstanding. There are some very quick wins in the safe domain and some very simple fixes that will improve outcomes and provide evidence that the care and treatment you provide is safe.

Mortality

The most important issue for people using services is around their mortality. There's not much use offering six flavours of ice cream if people are suffering from avoidable harm and even death.

In 2017, there were more than 140,000 (almost one in four) deaths that could have been averted or delayed through timely, effective healthcare and which were therefore considered avoidable. Cancers were the leading cause, followed by cardiovascular diseases, injuries, respiratory diseases and drug misuse.

This statistic is relevant to all health and social care practitioners, all practitioners in physical or mental health services, all grades of staff.

- In 2018, there were 6,507 suicides registered in the UK.
- In 2018, of all deaths among children and young people aged 0 to 19 years in the UK, 1,720 deaths out of 4,883 were considered avoidable.
- In 2010 there were 2,843 deaths from falls (excluding falls on building sites, ladders or off cliffs).
- In 2013 data shows 11,458 avoidable deaths related to infections, 40,805 related to cancers, and 11,745 related to respiratory disease.
- There were 18,765 avoidable deaths related to injuries in 2013.

It's not difficult to think of examples where people have died unnecessarily and it's very easy to see how, while the provider remains accountable for safe practice, individuals can do their part to reduce the risk of people dying unnecessarily.

An elderly patient died after drinking cleaning fluid because it was in a water jug on the ward. It is very easy in hindsight to think it couldn't happen to us, but I've been around several hospitals subsequently and seen the same cleaning fluid out on cleaning trolleys, on elderly care and children's wards. It was an acute hospital trust; it could just as easily been a care home or psychiatric unit.

Thinking about your role, your organisation, what can you do to reduce avoidable harm or death? Have you ever wondered whether you missed something or felt that you could have done something differently and prevented someone becoming more unwell or having an accident? Be honest with yourself here; it's hard but then think what you learned from those feelings and reflection.

If it helps, I'll tell you one that has lived with me. We had bought an old VW campervan for our foster son's amusement and because we couldn't afford a villa in Santorini. We spent many weekends camping, which, with a toddler and being pregnant, wasn't always very easy. We were in Bath to visit my in-laws and we'd set up the tent alongside the van, I'd set up the kitchen, fetched water and sorted supper and became increasingly irritated with my husband for a reason I can no longer remember. To appease me slightly, our foster son made a mug of tea for me and told me to sit down with it and relax for a while. The tea was far, far too hot to drink, so I put it beside the tiny camping stool I was perched on. Because I was heavily pregnant, I suddenly needed to go off to the lavatory. Our 21-month-old daughter was playing very happily on the grass but stumbled slightly and landed with her hand in my scalding tea. I heard the shriek from the shower block. We did the essential first aid of cold water and an ice pack wrapped in a tea towel, but it was clearly needing more. It healed over a few weeks with frequent dressings and she only has a very slight scar now, which you have to search for to spot. My husband and I felt so awful: it was entirely preventable, had I only stopped and thought. Had I asked for help with cooking instead of being a martyr to wifedom and motherhood, or had I formally passed over responsibility for our daughter's safety, she wouldn't have been injured. I still happily drink lukewarm tea, as that is what I became used to from then on.

Now back to your incident and where you could have acted in a different way or made a different decision and prevented harm. It doesn't have to be preventing a death, it's about preventing an accident or harm occurring. What was it, what do you wish you had done differently and what have you done since to stop it happening again?

Thinking about avoidable death and the leading causes, what do you or your team do well already to reduce the number of people dying prematurely? Do you do anything that is 'above and beyond' the norm for your type of service? Be specific! How well does your practice support early identification of risk and how well do you react when there is an elevated risk? What do you do really well?

Incidents

When I trained, we didn't have electronic incident reporting systems at all; the last slide rule was manufactured when I was doing A levels. My children wouldn't recognise it as a mathematical tool, but I think I could still use one.

When we messed up, we disappeared to the sluice, splashed our faces, tucked our hair in a bit more neatly under our caps, took a deep breath and came out to knock on Sister's door. It was scary but not quite as scary as being caught out, having not owned up. Even then we were encouraged to tell the truth and to own up to mistakes. We might have been told off very firmly, we might have to go and explain to the patient or parent, we had put things right as best we could, and we were expected to learn from our mistakes. So far, so good. I made mistakes and I learned.

What didn't happen was learning from other people's mistakes. I wasn't aware of any real trend analysis or identification of patterns of care lapses. Mortality was an expectation and not really considered on an individual basis; it was a very sad but deeply personal thing. It wasn't until 2001 that Dr Foster published its first *Hospital Guide* in the Sunday Times; it included mortality data using the Hospital Standardised Mortality Ratio (HSMR) for every hospital.

Incident review and analysis is still a relatively new science. Electronic reporting has moved on swiftly in many sectors but, as late as 2013, I recall working through an independent hospital's paper-based incident reports in a series of lever arch files to find evidence for enforcement action.

So, are we now better at learning from our mistakes and those of others? This is a really important area to reflect on and is key to services on their journey towards improved ratings.

Do you think it is important to report near misses and incidents and if so, why? What is your threshold for reporting? Who is responsible for reporting incidents in your area of practice? Would you change that?

What was the last incident or near miss you reported? How did you report it and what action was taken to reduce the risk of it happening again? If you can't think of one or have never reported an incident, why might that be?

Who provided you with feedback or discussion about the incident you reported? Who gave you the feedback or did you have to ask? Did you ask, if not told automatically and what was the response? Are you usually interested in the outcome?

Can you think of any incident that happened in your organisation that you weren't involved in? What was it and what action was taken? How did you find out about it? If it was in a newsletter or email, do you read those? Was there an opportunity for discussion and thinking about how it might affect your area of practice?

Why do you think some people are reluctant to report incidents and near misses? What stops them reporting using the providers process for incidents? What do you think happens to those incident reports, if anything? How does your organisation respond to you reporting incidents or raising concerns? Do you think the response might differ depending on who reported an incident? Could you report someone senior who made a mistake? What is the right thing to do?

How do you think reporting incidents impacts on inspection outcomes? Is it better to report lots of incidents or a few incidents? Does it make a difference what those incidents are or whether anyone was harmed, do you think? Is it more important to report everything or to just report the serious things and see if there are patterns? Why do you think as you do?

Can you think of any change you, your team or your organisation have because an incident was reported?

Individual risk assessments and care plans

This section isn't about environmental risk assessments, such as legionella risks or fire safety risk assessments. It's about individual risk assessments that inform care planning and delivery. You might call them something different, but the idea is the same. You consider the risks (or barriers) to each person's health and well-being, you think about what can be done to reduce the risks and promote good health and well-being and then you implement the agreed plan. This is where a care pathway for day surgery might sit – where most of the pathway is pre-determined but where there should still be consideration of individual needs. It's where a ReSPECT End of Life care document might sit and its where a woman's birth plan would sit.

It's much like cooking for a supper party – you think about what you want to cook with consideration of each guest's food likes and dislikes (what healthy looks like for this person), you think about what you need and what you don't have in the larder or fridge (the barriers and risks), then you write a shopping list that ensures you have all the necessary ingredients (care plan). Your crab tian, beef wellington and rhubarb parfait are only going to impress your guests if you actually go to the shop and buy the missing ingredients, then use them to cook with. That final bit is what the risk assessment and care planning process is about, it's the delivery of care based on the action plan that is important – taking the right action to improve someone's health and well-being.

From CQC website (provider information)
Key lines of enquiry

Are comprehensive risk assessments carried out for people who use services and risk management plans developed in line with national guidance? Are risks managed positively? How do staff identify and respond appropriately to changing risks to people, including deteriorating health and well-being, medical emergencies or behaviour that challenges? Are staff able to seek support from senior staff in these situations?

Something that has lived with me for a long time is a care home where there was a comprehensive personal risk assessment, giving details about the support and specialist equipment that a frail elderly man with advanced Parkinson's disease needed. It was regularly reviewed and updated; an exemplar of what a risk assessment and care plan should look like. Unfortunately, it wasn't enacted, and staff didn't use it as anything but a file to fill the office. The man suffered severe scalds because he was given near-boiling soup in an open bowl and he tipped it into his lap when trying to eat. I wince still when I picture his entirely avoidable injuries.

A risk assessment is a tool just as much as a hoist or a bread knife is a tool. It has a single purpose, which is to help staff identify the needs of a person in a structured way to ensure that no specific requirement or support is overlooked. In itself it is meaningless; just bits of paper or a computer file.

A good, holistic individual risk assessment tool should be eminently useable. If it's too complex or too wordy, it won't be completed properly. If it's not completed properly, or fully, the next inspection report will say something like, "There were individual risk assessments for each person, but there was inconsistency in how these were completed".

That may well then impact on your rating and instead of a lovely green or turquoise ratings grid, you might well have clusters of amber. Sadly, that inconsistency might simply be that a signature is missing from the seventh page or the allergies aren't listed for the fifth time on each section of the tool.

Think about how you assess a person's needs and preferences and how you document them. What is good about the risk assessments and care plans that you use in your organisation? How do you ensure they are current and reflect any changes in a person's needs or wishes? Who contributes to them? How much thought goes into completing them and do you involve the person the form is about?

Are there any ways they could be improved? Are they simple to use and completed fully? If not, what are the barriers that stop people filling them in properly? What could be done by you, your team or the organisation to ensure that they are seen as useful tools which are valued by staff?

Quick wins

There are many quick wins that can be accomplished and which motivate a team to greater success by building a positive 'can-do' culture. Too often time is spent in long meetings that achieve very little and which run the risk of disengaging staff – the exact opposite of what the organisation wants to achieve.

Quick wins can be introduced by individuals, by a team and by the organisation. If staff feel empowered to make suggestions and the leaders listen then much can be achieved very quickly.

Go back to thinking about first impressions. If a GP surgery has a door you can't see through because it is covered in scruffy out-of-date posters and badly written signs with curling edges, it is not going to give a good impression to anyone visiting. A quick win might be to buy a display board and ask someone to take responsibility for keeping it looking fresh, relevant and current. There is a bonus to the quick win – someone says how helpful the display on local services for people with diabetes is, so the owner of the display feels good about their work and makes even more effort. The manager who asked them to take on the responsibility feels good and sees that they can trust them to take on additional tasks. Quick wins and small successes are about more than just the quick win.

What areas of your practice do you think could be made better very easily? Have you ever thought, "If only someone did X or Y it would be better"? Are there times when you've had an idea that might make life easier or better but not shared it? What might the barriers be?

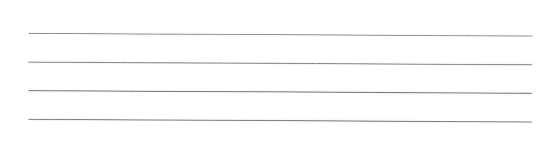

Taking five minutes to save an hour

Often, we say things like, "If only someone did X, it would save me hours". I'm sure we've all bemoaned not having enough time to do things properly both in our personal lives and in our professional roles. There are a myriad of ways to reduce wasted or inefficient use of time.

I'm not naturally the world's most organised person but, when the children were young I had a three-week menu (with some degree of flexibility) with a standard shopping list set out in groups, in the right order, as I went around the supermarket. I moved it to a standard online list as soon as online shopping became readily available. No time wasted thinking about meals or what I needed to make them. Nobody in the family spotted it was repetitive until I delegated the task of ordering the food to them when they were in their teens.

When I became a ward sister, I had my waist-length hair chopped to shoulder length. It saved a lot of time putting it up each day and, as a bonus, I was far more comfortable without a head full of pins weighed down by a huge plaited lump at the back of my head.

My daughter has just shown me a quick tip for the keyboard. My current favourite is Ctrl Z which will undo my last mistake. She likes to highlight then Shift F3 to change effortlessly between lower case and capitals. Saves time when writing an essay or slide show, as you just do everything lower case and then capitalise the bits you need to at the end.

I once watched staff in a care home approach each person who was sitting in the garden to ask whether they'd like an ice lolly. That was lovely on a warm summer day. They then went to the kitchen after each person responded and brought out one ice lolly before approaching the next person and repeating the trip to the kitchen. I asked why they didn't simply bring the lollies out and go round with them; they said they might melt. That was thoughtful but left me wondering why they hadn't got a cool box and ice packs.

In your place of work or in your role, can you think of any ways you could reduce the feeling of being constantly rushed? Where is time wasted? Are things left undone that would, if others took a few minutes, make life easier? It might be something as simple as having a notepad and pens beside each computer or it might be asking 'the friends' to purchase enough stethoscopes to avoid staff having to wander around the bays in search of one. It might be putting up clocks in rooms to reduce overrunning meetings; it could be standing handovers to avoid chit chat and to stay focused. For GPs it might be putting administration time in after every four patients; for an outpatient department it could be investing in pagers so that people didn't get grumpy when their clinic was running late; they could go off and have a cup of tea and be called back nearer the actual time they might be seen – thus saving staff time explaining and apologising. What are your ideas?

How could you put your ideas into practice?

_____

_____

_____

_____

_____

_____

Basic care as a quick win

There are some quite simple ideas that have blossomed and been shared across many services. I firmly believe in the value of simple things. If someone can't give a simple explanation of why something is important using everyday language, then they don't understand what they are trying to explain.

Basic care is an incredibly valuable quick win. Get this right and you will prevent avoidable deaths, pain and distress, loss of independence, hospital bed occupancy days, staff stress and sickness, loss of staff and money.

Mouthcare Matters

Mouthcare Matters is an initiative that started in East Surrey Hospital and which has spread across healthcare services through Health Education England. More details are in the main text that this journal is supplementary to, but the name almost says it all.

Good mouthcare makes a significant contribution to overall health and well-being. People with good oral health find eating easier, find speaking easier and can socialise without discomfort or embarrassment. It's impact is wide and good oral health can help reduce the incidents of pressure damage by supporting good nutrition and hydration; it can reduce the risk of urinary tract infections and acquired catheter infections and even potentially impact on the distressed behaviours of someone living with dementia.

Hospitalisation is associated with a deterioration of oral health in patients. This in turn has been linked to an increase in infections such as pneumonia, longer hospital stays and increased costs.

Good oral health is also important for patient safety, dignity and the ability to communicate, and is a key element of compassionate care.

I would recommend you spent some time looking at the Mouthcare Matters Website: https://mouthcarematters.hee.nhs.uk/

Thinking about yourself or your family members, how important is good oral health to you? Why is it important or unimportant? How do you ensure you maintain good oral health?

Do you visit the dentist regularly? Do you brush and floss regularly? Have you considered cosmetic dentistry such as teeth whitening or veneers? How comfortable are you smiling widely? How would you feel if someone said you had very bad breath? Is it even something that's OK to say? Do you carry peppermints, chewing gum or use a spray between brushing to avoid bad breath? Have you ever had toothache, an abscess, oral thrush or mouth ulcers?

How do you help the people you work with maintain good oral health? What are you good at? Is it even relevant to your area of work?

It might not be applicable to every consultation or every service, but there are a surprising number of situations where oral health should be considered. I'm thinking a travel clinic might just want to ask whether the person's travel insurance covers emergency dental treatment, for example. Maybe in an oncology clinic, or as a GP caring for people undergoing chemotherapy, you might think about prescribing an analgesic mouthwash to patients, so they had something to ease the discomfort of sore mouths. You might also want to give advice about which foods patients are more likely to taste and want to eat (cold beer being nicer than wine, for example).

Where do you get your oral health advice from? Do you have the skills and knowledge to support people's oral health or is it just assumed you know what brushing teeth is about? Are you given any advice where someone isn't able to take responsibility for their own mouth care? What if they simply don't want to bother; do you just let them decide or do you know of other strategies to reduce the impact of poor oral hygiene? Does your organisation have a policy, and have you seen it?

How could oral health be better supported in your place of work?

Do you think consideration of oral health can indicate a safeguarding concern? When might you share concerns?

_____

_____

_____

_____

There are lots of other areas of care that could theoretically be 'quick wins' on any improvement journey towards excellence, and hopefully an improved rating at the next inspection. I would reiterate that keeping the focus on the provision of outstanding care and treatment is far more important than aiming for an improved rating.

Mindfulness for Medicines

One area where there is often room for improvement is around medicines management. In March 2017, the World Health Organisation launched its Global Patient Safety Challenge: Medication Without Harm, with the aim of reducing severe avoidable medication-related harm globally by 50% over the following five years.

NHS Improvement tell us that there are an estimated 237 million 'medication errors' per year in the NHS in England. Adverse drug reactions which are definitely avoidable cost £98.5 million annually, contribute to 1,700 deaths and are directly responsible for approximately 700 deaths per year.

When prescribing or administering medicines there is a need to get it right first time, every time. There are reams and reams written about medicines management, professional guidance and legislation. All are important and the relevant details should be known and understood by those they apply to. Electronic prescribing undoubtedly reduces errors and is rolled out in many services, but they don't stop someone picking up the wrong bottle or confusing the chart for Mrs Davison with that for Mrs Davidson, when in a rush.

Mindfulness is a technique which involves making a special effort to notice what's happening in the present moment (in your mind, body and surroundings). It is being aware of what is happening in the here and now. It can reduce medicines errors, among other benefits. Being mindful of what you are giving to whom and when doesn't sound very complicated, but we often get it wrong, sometimes with disastrous consequences.

Taking it right back to first principles really does reduce the risk of errors, and we were taught that immediately before handing over any drugs that we should stop and ask ourselves whether it was:

- The right drug.
- The right dose.
- The right patient.
- The right time.
- The right route of administration.

Not complex, not overly burdensome to do in your everyday practice, and much safer and cheaper than giving Mrs Davison's oral Morphine Sulphate to Mrs Davies via an intravenous cannula.

That 'one-minute stop and think again' before administering the drug could save a life, prevent serious complications and preserve your professional registration. It's even more important to do when under pressure or acting in an emergency. Certainly, in some situations (and against good practice guidance) some services accept drugs being put out by a different person to the person administering them. This might be so that there is a more efficient flow through an operating theatre or because they know what the consultant in an outpatient department usually likes. I remember a time when I was working as an agency nurse in a nursing home in Surrey. I was surprised that the nursing assistant had made a bed up for me but horrified that she had put all the drugs out in little plastic cups with the room numbers written onto them. Her expectation was that I would simply sign the charts for her. She was aghast that I threw them all away and insisted on starting from scratch; it took much longer as I didn't know anyone, and the charts were not always very clear. That extra time didn't matter but the safety of the patients did: I was being paid to work a night shift not to sleep until morning.

How well do you stay focused when prescribing or administering drugs of any sort? How well informed are you about the professional requirements and laws around medicines? How well do you, your team and your organisation follow the requirements? How neat and legible are your drug records? How much crossing out is there?

Have you ever made a mistake (or had a near miss) when prescribing or administering a drug? Most people working in health and social care have. What were the circumstances? Was there anything that could have prevented it? Was it reported? If so, what happened? How did you feel?

Findings from the review of deaths of patients at Gosport War Memorial Hospital between 1988 and 2000 showed that over 450 patients had died prematurely; many of these deaths were avoidable. There was an institutionalised culture of prescribing and administering 'dangerous doses' of a combination of drugs which were not clinically indicated or justified.

Are you aware of any poor practice that falls outside the national guidance or your organisation's policy for safe medicines management? For example, pre-drawing up, little cups of sedation medicines on bedside cabinets in care homes, not having two people check controlled drugs, sharing of individually prescribed medicines or using the same vial for different patients. Maybe think about drug storage or who has access to stock. What have you done about this?

What do you do if you are uncertain about something to do with medicines? Who do you ask? Who could you ask? What sources of information are there to check that the prescription is appropriate if your instincts are telling you that something isn't right?

Are you confident with drug calculations, if necessary? Do you know the usual dosage range of common drugs for your work role? What might be triggers for you to question the prescription (or what you were about to prescribe)? Have you ever felt a pressure to prescribe or administer a drug when you have felt it wasn't the right thing to do without checking? What would you do?

It is estimated that every day about 35,000 people with learning disabilities or autism are prescribed drugs that affect their mental state when they do not have a diagnosed mental health condition. This is often done to manage behaviour which is seen as challenging. It includes medicines used to treat psychosis, depression, anxiety and sleep disorders. It also includes epilepsy drugs given to people who do not have epilepsy, to calm them.

Chemical restraint is the use of medication which is prescribed and administered for the purpose of controlling or subduing disturbed/violent behaviour, where it is not prescribed for the treatment of a formally identified physical or mental illness. It is sometimes seen when a service is caring for people living with dementia, as well as in services for people with learning disabilities. Sometimes people are automatically given sleeping drugs so that they are less likely to ask for assistance at night.

How do you view the use of drugs to calm people? Would you see it as a Deprivation of Liberty or a safeguarding concern? Might chemical restraint breach the Equalities Act (2010)? Have you seen chemical restraint used? What alternatives could be tried? Staff should look for other causes of distressed behaviour before using chemical restraint. What might those causes be? What strategies might be effective?

Part 3:
Is it effective?

Introduction

The Commission website says, "There are five questions we ask of all care services. They're at the heart of the way we regulate, and they help us to make sure we focus on the things that matter to people." The effective domain is about outcomes, competent staff, following national guidance and benchmarking services. It incorporates nutrition, pain management, consent and multi-disciplinary working.

Effective: your care, treatment and support achieve good outcomes, helps you to maintain quality of life and is based on the best available evidence

Characteristics of services we would rate as outstanding in this area are where outcomes for people who use services are consistently better than expected when compared with other similar services.

Nutrition and hydration

From the inspection framework

How are people's nutrition and hydration needs (including those related to culture and religion) identified, monitored and met? Where relevant, what access is there to dietary and nutritional specialists to assist in this?

While this might logically be considered under the Safe key question, in the CQC framework it sits under the Effective key question. Poor nutrition and hydration most certainly impacts on patient safety in terms of pressure damage, wound healing, infection risk and acute kidney injury, but it is wider.

The framework suggests it is not applicable to dentists, GP practices or GP Out-of-Hours or NHS 111 services. It would be unreasonable to expect a dentist to do a full nutritional assessment, although poor nutrition impacts on oral health and, thus, is relevant to dentistry. Similarly, nutrition is something that is of relevance to a GP service – although not necessarily as a full nutritional assessment at every appointment.

For most services however, food and drink are very important. As we age, we stop replacing taste buds and those we have shrink making us likely to have reduced sense of taste as we enter old age. To maintain the pleasure in mealtimes, good food is necessary that is both nice to look at and which smells good.

I think many well-intentioned staff and services think older people won't like strong tastes, spicy or 'modern' foods. I've certainly been in a few places where I've been offered lunch; what I rejected was an unidentifiable plate of greyish mush. It was probably poached fish with mashed potatoes or chicken in a white sauce with rice, I'll never know, but just hope nobody serves me similar in my dotage. Many older people I know (think octogenarians) like a curry or burger, as much as the next person. That bit about Mouthcare Matters comes into its own here. It is grossly unfair to take away the joy of food from people because of ill-fitting dentures that make their mouth sore. Good food gets eaten. Good food results in better health. Good food reduces pressure damage. Good food brings pleasure and offers a topic for conversation, when life itself is limited.

There is some incredible food being provided in some services. Often, hospices lead the way along with good care homes. NHS hospital food is more of a challenge because they are catering for so many on such limited budgets, but things can be done if one thinks outside the box.

When our son had suffered a head injury playing rugby and was admitted to our local hospital for a couple of days, he was told he could go home after he'd had something to eat. He, like his father, believes hospitals are germ-ridden places with pathogenic bacteria, waiting to colonise him, hiding in every nook and cranny. He simply refused to eat anything at all that was purchased, made or heated in the hospital. A wise paediatrician told us to order an extra-large pepperoni pizza and an extra-large margherita pizza, from a national chain, and have it delivered to the ward. We explained that, while he had a very healthy appetite usually, even a teenage boy wouldn't manage two extra-large deep pan pizzas. She was clear that if he saw others looking on with envy and he sniffed the familiar smell of a pizza, he'd feel much better and eat quite happily; he simply wasn't given to eating lukewarm cod in cheese sauce. The 'two extra-large' was because what he didn't eat the staff would appreciate... It was about consideration of personal and cultural norms.

What are your food needs and preferences? How important is food to you? Is it just 'fuel for the body' or is it also 'fuel for the soul'? How fussy are you? Do you have particular needs and are these the same as preferences? Do you enjoy cooking? Do you treat yourself with food at all? How often? Do you prefer to eat alone or with friends? What would your 'last meal' be? Do mealtimes give you pleasure? What about drinks throughout the day, what do you like?

Is there anything you really can't bring yourself to eat? For me it's jellied eels. Are there things that put you off eating a meal before or during the meal? When would you send a restaurant meal back? Do you eat all your food at set mealtimes, or do you snack?

_____

What do you or your team do particularly well regarding food? How personal are the food choices? How much variety is there? How do you encourage people to eat and drink? What about snacks or missed meals (what is, theoretically, on offer and what is actually made available)? Would you eat the food? How do you support people who find eating and drinking difficult? What expert help do you have access to and how often is it used? Do you go the 'extra mile' and if so in what way?

_____

How would you feel about being fed? What might it feel like from a psychological and a physical perspective? What might you dislike about it? Would you prefer to be fed in a communal area or with privacy? Does being unable to hold a cup mean you prefer lukewarm tea? Would you still fancy an ice-cold beer or an ice lolly on a warm day or would you want to minimise the number of times you needed to be fed?

_____

If you were supporting someone to eat, how could you improve the experience? Think about staffing, setting, conversation, speed, choice, utensils, taste and temperature.

_____

_____

_____

_____

_____

How good is the food that is served where you work? What is good about it and what could be improved? Are people asked to give feedback on the food? What do they say? Are they asked for ideas of what they might like? Are the cooks or chefs told about feedback? Do they ever talk to people who use the service about food? If there is a complaint about food are the catering staff made aware of it? If someone just wants pudding, can they have two portions? Do some people just get 'what there is' – for example, does ice cream often run out on your ward? What is breakfast like? What options are there for snacks?

_____

_____

_____

_____

_____

How can people get treats, snacks or replacement meals? Can they have a take-away or have a ready meal heated in a microwave? Can family members bring meals to be heated up? Are people told they can go to the shop or on-site café? Would staff help them?

_____

_____

_____

_____

_____

How easy is it to get a drink between meals (that isn't water)? What range of drinks is on offer? Can people bring their own teabags or coffee? Is a barista coffee available or could it be? Is ice available for squash or juice and is it offered? Could people have a mug rather than a tiny cup of tea and saucer? How could people get a cola or other fizzy drink? Do you use drinks for nutritional support by making creamy milkshakes or smoothies from fresh fruit? If not, why not?

What is your organisational policy on the consumption of alcohol? What are the risks of alcohol consumption for the people you work with (I don't mean other staff)? How would you balance risk from alcohol against personal freedoms? Would you put beer in the fridge for a person using your services? Would you set limits on what or how much alcohol could be consumed (e.g. a sherry or small beer is OK, but half a bottle of wine isn't)? Do you have a right to set limits?

How do you encourage and support healthy eating? Does the food your service provides contain sufficient vegetables? How often is fruit offered as a snack? How do you approach someone who is obese but wanting lots of high calorie food or drinks? Do you have a discussion or not? Why do you think it matters if they are very elderly and fat? If you work in surgery or are a commissioner, how honest are you about the low risk of anaesthesia even if you are overweight?

Obesity is a risk factor for postoperative complications in general surgery. Research in the BMC Anesthesiology by Elke, Sanne, Hoeks *et al* concluded that:

> *"Obesity alone is a significant risk factor for wound infection, more surgical blood loss and a longer operation time. However, being obese is associated with improved long-term survival, validating the obesity paradox. We also found that complication and mortality rates are significantly worse for underweight patients. Our findings suggest that a tendency to regard obesity as a major risk factor in general surgery is not always justified. It is the underweight patient who is most at risk of major postoperative complications, including long-term mortality."*

What do you think when you read this? Are people refused surgery based on prejudice or cost alone? Should we be encouraging people to put on weight to live longer? What does healthy look like? Controversial!

Pain

Chronic pain is suffered by over a third of the population. It is often distressing and can be disabling; many cannot work and lose their jobs.

Treatment of pain is a fundamental human right, yet sadly there is an enormous gap between the care people require and what happens in practice. Sometimes people don't have the words to describe pain. Sometimes pain is exhibited as distress, anger, moodiness, laziness or introversion. Recognising pain is the first step to preventing or treating it.

How would you define pain? We all think we know what it means, but how do you put that into words? Are there different sorts of pain? Does pain affect different people in different ways?

_____

_____

_____

_____

_____

_____

Pain is defined by the British Pain Society as:

> *"An emotion experienced in the brain, it is not like touch, taste, sight, smell or hearing. It is categorised into Acute pain - less than twelve weeks duration and Chronic pain - of more than twelve weeks. Pain can be perceived as a warning of potential damage but can also be present when no actual harm is being done to the body."*

Often there is an obvious cause of pain: if we stub our toe or graze our knee it is clear why there is pain. There are times however, when the reason for pain is not obvious and there are no clear physical symptoms. Many will have woken up with stiff legs after running a long-distance race or driving all day. There are no symptoms apart from the reported pain and stiffness but nobody would doubt it was real.

Pain can be a warning sign that something more serious is wrong. It can help the body know to rest or seek advice.

We respond instinctively to pain sometimes. Which parent or grandparent hasn't rubbed something better? Rubbing a sore knee or arm after a bump really does help make the pain go away. Gentle stroking activates 'pleasure' nerves beneath the skin, which then reduce the sensation of pain from other nerves. People who were exposed to painful temperatures on the surface of their skin felt less pain if they were stroked at the same time. This might well resonate with parents who have stroked their child's back while they have an injection or when they are unwell with an ear infection. It is believed that signals to the brain from the nerves that detect the pleasurable stroking dampen the signals from nerves that detect pain.

Can you remember when you have felt the most pain in your life? Are you able to describe it and the circumstances? How did it affect you? What did you do to try and ease the pain? How well did this work? Did it affect how you responded to other people?

Many factors affect and impact on our perception of pain including:

- Attention. Paying too much attention to a painful stimulus can increase the intensity. Distraction is a good analgesic.

- Expectations. A person's experience of a specific pain can affect the reaction to the same exposure in the future. This is hugely important to understand if you work with children. A poor prior experience and lack of comfort can override normal feedback from pain receptors, turning what should be a mild pain into a severe one.

- Interpretation. How we self-assess a pain varies according to the context. Someone who had previously suffered a heart attack, for example, may fixate on an irrelevant muscle ache in their ribs and blow it out of all proportion.

- Context. A hockey player about to score a goal who is hit with a stick may barely notice the pain amidst the excitement of the game. A person getting hit with the same force in the street by an unknown assailant may experience a much higher level of pain.

- Emotions. Fear, anxiety, depression and general distress can increase our perception of pain. Someone who has had cancer may feel a backache as far more intense than someone who has not had cancer. People with depression, for example, are more likely to seek help for pain.

There are many examples where people undergoing similar procedures report very different levels of pain. The reason isn't always clear, and it isn't necessarily about who is brave and who 'makes a fuss'. Certainly, a sound understanding of what is happening reduces the level of fear and consequently the reaction to any discomfort.

A clear example of this would be very different experiences of women undergoing hysteroscopy. The Campaign Against Painful Hysteroscopy is a group of UK patients who have had hysteroscopies and who are concerned that a sizeable minority (5%-25%) of UK hysteroscopy patients have reported severe pain during these outpatient procedures. They believe that their pain was so significant that all women should be offered a choice of general anaesthetic. The other 75% of patients report little or no pain above mild cramping. The usual advice is to take paracetamol an hour beforehand.

When you think about the pain which you described, do you think any of the factors mentioned above had an impact?

Why do you think the pain felt so bad? Why do you think some women feel the need for a general anaesthetic whereas some are fine with a couple of paracetamol capsules?

A study by Peacock and Patel in 2008 published in the *British Journal of Pain* concluded that ethnic minority communities are at a disadvantage regarding treatment for painful conditions. It is demonstrated that people from ethnic groups receive less provision of preventative healthcare, provision of medication and secondary referrals than host nationals.

What do you think the reasons for this might be? What do you think could be done to address the issue locally and nationally?

Now think about your own practice. How do you assess pain? Do you simply ask people if they have pain? Do you ask them to score their pain? What if people can't tell you about the type or intensity of their pain (babies, children, people lacking cognition, people unable to give a verbal response, people who speak another language)? Do you consider behavioural changes as potentially indicative of pain? What do you do well and what could you do better?

What do you offer to address people's pain? Do you simply offer drugs, or do you have a broader repertoire to help ease pain? Is your response to pain timely? Do you encourage people to use drugs to prevent pain, or only provide analgesia when requested? Do you offer advice on coping strategies or methods of reducing pain?

Would you 'allow' the use of hot water bottles or heating pads? If not, why not? Do you base your practice on evidence or intuition?

From January 2008 to September 2009, there were only two admissions to hospital following hot water bottle burns in Australia. However, a research study by Anglia Ruskin University, reviewed on the ITV website, examined the notes of 50 patients with burns from hot water bottle use between January 2004 and February 2012. In eight of the cases there was some degree of patient misuse, such as sitting or stepping on the bottle. In the remaining 17 cases there was no clear evidence of misuse and the bottle appeared to have burst spontaneously. Accidental spilling of hot water while filling a hot water bottle accounted for 32% of injuries, with the remaining 18% due to contact with an excessively hot surface.

Does the evidence change your view at all? If you would consider the use of hot water bottles or heat pads, what limitations would you put on their use? What safety measures might you put in place? If you do not provide direct care, would you recommend a hot water bottle?

The British Journal of Nursing published an online research article, 'Parental presence and distraction during painful childhood procedures' by Matziou _et al_. The cohort was children aged 7–10 years and the results showed that children who had their parent close to them showed a reduction in breathing rate, blood pressure and pulse compared to the children whose parents were absent. They also felt less pain and they were less distressed.

As a paediatric nurse this comes as no surprise. It seems all too obvious. If a child is distressed or hurt, they usually run to a parent or other loving and trusted adult. We recognise this and parents are actively encouraged to remain with their child when they are in a hospital setting. Parents remain with their child while they are anaesthetised and should be called to recovery as soon as possible.

When does this calming and reducing effect stop working? I know I was permitted into the operating theatre at our local hospital with our son when he had an emergency appendectomy in the middle of the night. He was 17, certainly not a tiny child, but still frightened and in pain.

How would you feel about an adult having a relative or friend remain with them in the anaesthetic room or during another invasive procedure? Why? Would it make a difference if the person had dementia, didn't speak the same language as you or was particularly anxious? Would you offer it or wait to be asked? Is this a view or is it evidence-based?

Learning and competence

If you've got this far through the journal, you either enjoy learning, have a natural curiosity and desire to understand or you have been made to participate. I hope the former, but if your service leaders are encouraging learning and reflection, then that is also a good thing. Hopefully, you will still find something in it that makes you think or want to understand more.

You cannot be an outstanding organisation or an excellent staff member without a commitment to learning. That learning can take many forms, from watching a television documentary, to talking with peers or hearing someone's personal story. It doesn't need to be about completing e-learning or gaining formal qualifications. We should all learn something (or indeed many things) every day – it keeps life interesting and means we know what's going on. Today, for example, I learned that the UK only has one city that begins with the letter K and that it's not usually known by that name. Thank you to Richard Osman and his lockdown weekly quiz that I do with my daughter. I suspect you'll now need to go and have a think or use a search engine.

We need to maintain professional competence and make sure our knowledge and skills remain current, but hopefully we'll want to go above and beyond that in all aspects of our life.

One thing I've set up since lockdown is to host a professional reading group. It's been really nice to step outside of all things Coronavirus for an hour and focus on something in an informal and non-hierarchical setting. The house rules are that people can have opinions that oppose each other's, or the majority view, but they must then be open to challenge and not be hurtful to others. We take and read a national report or piece of guidance then discuss it, as simple as that. The Mid-Staffordshire Inquiry report, the Morecombe Bay Inquiry report, the Child Health report from the Royal College of Paediatrics and Child Health have all featured. We discuss the issues that are raised and think about how this impacts on our work. The conversation is unstructured and can take us off at all sorts of tangents, we share experiences and stories and hopefully learn something along the way. It's fun, it's light, but it is also important that we understand the recommendations from those reports. People engage at a level they are comfortable with. Some want detailed technical answers to their questions, others want to consider the ethical issues it raises.

I'm not personally a fan of 'one size fits all training'. I accept it has a place and that there are areas that all staff need to learn about, but we all come from such different levels of prior experience and knowledge that what may be overly complicated for some is too basic to engage others. I think reflective practice offers opportunities for that differentiation.

What sorts of things have you learned (big or small, personal or professional) in the past week?

Think about something you have really enjoyed learning. What was it and why was it so good?

How do you find the training you are provided with, or lead, in your organisation? Do you learn anything? Does it leave you wanting even more answers? What methods are used, and which do you prefer? How could it be improved?

While some required formal qualifications cannot be changed, developing competency and increasing the knowledge of your team can boost not only learning, but staff engagement, innovation and team-building. It can provide an opportunity for working together with a purpose.

What areas of your work would you like to know more about or understand better? What questions do you have? How might you find answers to those questions?

_____

_____

_____

_____

_____

_____

How could you share your skills and knowledge better within your organisation or part of the organisation? You might want to think outside the usual way of doing things.

_____

_____

_____

_____

_____

How might the following be received as potential ways of sharing learning? What are the advantages and disadvantages? Which do you think might be more powerful ways of sharing learning and improving care?

- Schwartz round style meetings focusing on stories about the impact of work on how individual staff feel and how they have found solutions to both the situation and the personal challenges.
- An email update about action taken after an incident was reported.
- A learning slot at a team meeting where someone presents an update on a specific issue such as syringe drivers or changes to NICE guidance.
- A study day with highly respected speakers, delivered in a lecture theatre.
- A multi-disciplinary (or single staff group) case study reflection, looking at the care of an individual (real or hypothetical) and discussing how the best care could be provided considering the person holistically.
- E-learning.

_____

_____

_____

_____

_____

_____

_____

_____

How could you improve the learning culture in your service or team? Is it even your responsibility to encourage learning?

_____

_____

_____

_____

_____

_____

_____

_____

How staff, teams and services work together

Characteristics of services CQC would rate as outstanding in this area (for healthcare)

Staff, teams and services are committed to working collaboratively and have found innovative and efficient ways to deliver more joined-up care to people who use services.

There is a holistic approach to planning people's discharge, transfer or transition to other services, which is done at the earliest possible stage.

Very rarely do services provide care or treatment in complete isolation from other teams or agencies. Very rarely does one professional group work without input from any other professionals. This is true whether you work in a care home, a service for people with learning disabilities, a specialist trust or a GP practice or a 111-call centre. We all need to forge positive professional relationships with others.

Who outside of your immediate team and professional discipline do you personally work with? Think inside your organisation and with other agencies and professionals. This isn't about relationships with the people using services or their relatives; it's about cross profession, cross team and cross agency working.

How would you say relationships were? Are they equal, respectful? Are they warm and encouraging of joint working? Are everyone's views respected? Are there any relationships that are less established or more challenging?

Can you think back to whether there has ever been a relationship with an individual that has been a bit tricky? How difficult was it and what was the impact on people using the service? It might be a real clash, or it might be they didn't really share information with you. You might have felt they were dismissive of your perspective or didn't follow best practice guidance. How did it present? How did it feel? Did you feel supported by your manager to address it?

Reflecting on how the situation came to be, and how it persisted over time, what do you think the important factors were? Was your reaction helpful or did it exacerbate the situation? Is there anything you would (or could) do differently if you had your time over again?

Thinking about relationships you see as working well, what do you think it is that makes it an effective and professional relationship?

How do you think you make it easier for people to have a good relationship with you? What personal qualities, professional knowledge and behaviours help develop relationships that are in the best interests of people using services? Then, conversely, is there anything about you that makes you less approachable or less likely to be involved in cross professional discussions?

In your organisation, what could be done to improve cross professional working – not necessarily only about personal relations but also about the effectiveness of the relationship? Are all professions and staff equal? Do the women make the tea? Would someone make tea and bring a biscuit for a junior doctor on medical take overnight who barely had time to breathe? Are maverick behaviours tolerated by the organisation's management? How does it work if one of the people who you perceive as challenging is a partner or leader? Would you be supported if you raised concerns? What are the barriers to improved working relations?

Can you think of how you could demonstrate good interprofessional and inter-agency working? What evidence could you present? How could you show that relationships were effective and that they improved outcomes?

Do you collate the evidence you receive or send feedback to others about your interactions? (This could be a thank you card to the GP that visits your care home regularly and always goes the extra mile, a note to the junior doctor who has stayed on the ward most of the night because they were concerned about a patient, or an email to the CCG about how well supported you feel). What could you do to make others feel good about their professional relationship with you? Do you tell colleagues when you have enjoyed working with them or learned something from them?

Mistakes often happen because of misunderstandings and one person not hearing or recalling fully what another professional had said. This might be something minor, but it can also be something significant.

I remember a friend returning to our shared house appalled because, when she was in charge of a neonatal unit overnight, an agency nurse had misheard or misunderstood the instruction to feed a baby 30mls of GEM via their tube. GEM is Glucose-Electrolyte Mixture which was used when feeding was being introduced after bowel surgery. Instead of checking, instead of looking at the feeding regime document, the nurse assumed she understood and pottered off to the kitchen. She was next seen when the ventilator alarm sounded. She had disconnected the machine and was attempting to spoon a small pot of strawberry jelly down the endotracheal tube into the baby's lungs. Luckily, the ventilator settings were set such that the alarms were triggered very quickly, and the baby was reconnected without any noticeable harm. It could have been a different outcome.

We were incredulous that anyone could have been so daft but then we knew the jargon of the hospital, we knew the normal regimes and we had English as our first language.

What systems do you have in your workplace to ensure misunderstandings or lapses of care due to miscommunication between visiting professionals don't affect patient safety and well-being? Are they used properly? If not, why not? How could they be improved?

Consent

What do you understand informed consent to mean? When do you seek consent? Is it applicable to your setting? Who is responsible for gaining consent? Who can give consent?

_____

_____

_____

_____

_____

_____

Thinking about how important autonomy and consent are to you, what are your thoughts on the following situations?

- Arranged marriages.
- Your partner booking a 'surprise' holiday to watch the Evian women's golf championships by secretly arranging for you to have five days leave and booking a caravan to share with another couple.
- Annual leave being allocated rather than requested.
- Your young adult or child uses your Amazon account to order a tent and other items for a festival.
- One person 'does the finances' and their partner is required to provide receipts for all expenses.
- A friend or neighbour lets themself into your house or flat and puts the kettle on as they can hear you are in the shower.
- A smoking and alcohol ban on all public beaches.

_____

_____

_____

_____

How would you feel if you had to ask to leave the house? Coronavirus lockdown has removed autonomy and control to varying degrees. How do you feel about not being able to visit friends or go to restaurants? How do you feel about families not being able to be together?

Assuming an adult patient, when can a doctor or healthcare professional withhold information to protect their person from distress? What if they aren't sure the person is ready for bad news? What if a person's family don't want them told they are dying or very unwell? Do you think relatives or spouses have a right to know and be involved in decision-making like this?

I suspect many of us have told 'white' lies. The majority of people lie in everyday conversation when they are trying to appear likable and competent. A study by Robert Feldman at the University of Massachusetts found that 60% of people lied at least once during a 10 minute conversation and told an average of two to three lies.

Have you ever withheld information from someone because you felt it might not be in their best interests, or told a lie to someone because you felt it was better for them – either in your personal life or professional life? What were the circumstances and what made you think it was better for the other person? How do you think they might have reacted if they knew you were lying or withholding information? Is honesty always best?

How much information do you give to people to help them decide? When is consent not informed? Is it then valid? Do you ever apply pressure (however well intentioned) to people when the decision is theirs to make? This might be small things like whether to wear a hat in the sun or it might be much more complex such as whether a person with mental health difficulties should abort a pregnancy.

Is the information you provide unbiased and sufficient? Do you perhaps strongly recommend a particular type of contraception by highlighting benefits and minimising risks, or might you talk a care home resident out of buying an electric tricycle?

This next question becomes very pertinent as I am writing in the middle of the Covid-19 pandemic and there are some very difficult decisions and conversations going on across the globe. The questions apply predominantly to the UK – other countries have different legislative requirements.

Can relatives or patients insist a medical team 'do everything possible' to give a 'fighting chance' of life? Can they insist on more chemotherapy, for example, or surgery for an obstructed bowel in a 96-year-old?

What about as someone approaches the end of their life, can they insist on continuing to be given active treatment such as chemotherapy if they retain capacity?

Do you know where the responsibility for these decisions falls and what legislation or national guidance it comes under? If you don't know, who do you think is responsible?

How well do you understand the Mental Capacity Act (2005)? I'm sure you have completed mandatory training around it, but what is your level of knowledge actually like? What do you think the key principles are? Clue: there are five. How important is it to uphold the principles?

Do you support or allow people to make unwise decisions? Or do you allow people to make decisions except ones you feel are too unwise? How does this work in practice? Would a patient think the 'doctor was cross with them' or the care home resident feel 'they weren't really allowed to'? Can you think of an unwise decision you have supported? How did that feel for you?

How often do you refer to people as 'lacking capacity' when handing over, talking to other staff or visiting professionals? In practice, how do you manage to ensure that the MCA is applied for each decision rather than as a blanket assessment that someone 'lacks capacity'?

How do you involve families in decision-making or update them about care and condition where people using your service are elderly? Do you automatically share information and discuss care or treatment with relatives and spouses? Do you expressly ask elderly people whether it's OK to talk to their relatives and spouses?

If someone has limited spoken English, how do you ensure that there is informed consent? What is your policy about translation and does practice mirror policy? How does this work in a small service, a GP practice or dental clinic? How do you ensure someone who uses sign language as their first language can give informed consent? How often do you use relatives to translate or do you rely on free internet translation? Are all written consent forms in English? Is it possible to get non-English, braille or other forms easily? If you are not using translation, how is consent informed? What could you, as a service, do to improve how well you gained consent?

If children under 18 years of age use your service, when can they give consent, do you think? What factors influence this? Do you accept consent from children in your service?

In 1983, the criteria were laid out for establishing whether a child under 16 has the capacity to provide consent to treatment; the so-called 'Gillick test'.

It was determined that children under 16 years of age can consent if they have sufficient understanding and intelligence to fully understand what is involved in a proposed treatment, including its purpose, nature, likely effects and risks, chances of success and the availability of other options.

How do you assess a child's ability to consent to a specific decision? Is it recorded, and is it compliant with the guidance? Do you assume that children understand fully the information you are giving them, or do you have some formal process for assessing their understanding of all the risks and possible alternatives?

How do you encourage children attending alone to involve their parents in decision-making? Is this recorded, is there an organisational policy about parental involvement in decision-making? How do you link this to considerations of safeguarding? How could you improve parental involvement in decision-making?

As a final reflection, imagine how you might feel if your opinion wasn't listened to and your decision was overruled? Imagine someone else deciding what you ate, what you wore, who you had to see and what activities you had to take part in, or which were not permitted. What would you find hardest?

Part 4:
Is it Caring?

Caring

Caring is something everyone understands, isn't it? We all like to think of ourselves as exceptionally caring and yet the most complaints about services are not around outcomes, are not about medicines errors or even ghastly food. They are about communication, staff attitude and a perceived lack of caring.

> By caring, we mean that the service involves and treats people with compassion, kindness, dignity and respect.
>
> Services that are rated as 'Outstanding' in this area are where people are truly respected and valued as individuals and are empowered as partners in their care, practically and emotionally, by an exceptional and distinctive service.

It's all a bit difficult to measure, isn't it? Providing evidence for the improvements in mortality rate or in the number of falls is easy. Showing that there is true respect or that people are empowered is a whole lot harder to demonstrate.
We probably all have different perceptions of what being caring means; the range of behaviours that people would describe as undignified varies enormously.

I found a couple of definitions of dignity:

- the state or quality of being worthy of honour or respect
- a composed or serious manner, or style or a sense of pride in oneself; self-respect.

Surely the first is true of everyone: people deserve respect. I'm not sure only the serious are dignified but perhaps enabling people to retain or develop a sense of pride in themselves is key to what we mean.

It's a purely personal view, but I think the Caring domain underpins all other key questions in the inspection framework. I know others would perhaps say that Safety is most important or that being Well-led is the key to excellence. My view is that if the organisational culture supports kindness and compassion then the rest is likely to follow. Truly caring staff bother about the small things and pay attention to detail, these add up to keep people safe and promote good outcomes.

If you care enough to notice Mrs Smith's glasses are covered in dried food and that her slippers are on the wrong feet, then if you are sufficiently kind to clean the glasses and swap the slippers around, Mrs Smith will be less likely to fall.

If you are kind and listen when Graham Collins wants to discuss his insomnia, he may open up about his company going into administration, long-serving employees losing their jobs and his wife leaving him. It might transpire that he has been struggling with thoughts of despair, and kindness might help determine the degree of risk he is at.

If you are kind when Carrie Jones comes to antenatal care and mentions that she is ambivalent about the pregnancy and a bit worried about how she'll cope, she might feel sufficiently supported to mention that her partner is violent when he's had a drink and she is frightened for her safety.

Please don't underrate how important kindness and compassion are as vital components of excellence.

Looking back, can you think of a time when someone has been particularly kind to you personally? It needn't be related to health or social care. What were the circumstances? What made it stand out as over and above what people usually do? How did it make you feel?

_____

_____

_____

_____

_____

Now think of a time when you have been particularly kind or caring to someone else. Not just a 'generally nice' sort of thing but something specific. What were the circumstances. Why did you decide to be particularly kind? What made it unusual? How did you show you cared? How did it make you feel?

_____

_____

_____

_____

_____

Finally, move to your work setting. When have you gone 'the extra mile'? What did you do that exceeded the usual expectations of kindness towards people using your service or another member of staff? Was it outside of your organisation's policy? Was it in your own time or at your own expense? How did you put yourself out for others?

How do the staff and leaders in your workplace, in your own team and across the organisation treat each other? Are you kind to each other? How does this work in practice? What do you do for each other that is more than everyday rubbing along together?

If your leaders, your co-workers and other professionals are nice to you, how does that impact on your mood and demeanour? Does this affect how you do your job and how you interact with others? If someone remembers your birthday with a card, are you more likely to smile at others? Do people offer to help others with their work or take on additional tasks to let people get away in good time?

How are lower grade staff treated? How do ward staff treat the junior doctors, care home owners treat the cook and Directors treat the cleaners?

I once had a minor procedure that was done very well with kind and attentive staff. I was asked to complete a questionnaire but, since it was handed to me with a cup of tea by a healthcare assistant, and I was the only person using the service at the time, it would have been quite hard to write anything negative as I was immediately identifiable. Thankfully I had no concerns, but while the process might have boosted their feedback scores, it rather inhibited the learning from feedback.

If having thought about it you believe you are an exceptionally kind and caring service, how could you demonstrate this? What evidence could you present and how? How do you measure compassion? Do you know whether people using the service think you are as caring as you think you are? If you use surveys in small organisations, how do you ensure they are anonymous, so that people feel they can provide feedback freely?

_____

_____

_____

_____

_____

_____

Key Line of Enquiry

Do staff understand and respect the personal, cultural, social and religious needs of people and how these may relate to care needs, and do they take these into account in the way they deliver services? Is this information recorded and shared with other services or providers?

We all have a perception of what good care looks like and the risk is we impose this on others.

I was leading a virtual professional reading group a couple of weeks ago and a question came up about whose view of what good care looked like was the most valid when inspecting – the inspection team's or the person using services? It was an interesting discussion about social norms, professional expectations and where these might conflict with individual preferences. We questioned whether a very overweight, elderly person who had what we considered a very poor diet of jelly babies, sherry, digestive biscuits with cream cheese and bananas would come under pressure to eat a bit more healthily? If that were what a care home resident was eating, would we be critical of the home? I'm not sure we agreed an answer.

Do you have any personal, social, cultural, or religious needs or simply things that are important to you? Think about food, clothes, activities, music, hygiene and personal grooming, pets, family. What would you not want to change, where are your red lines? What would the perfect service for you look like?

How well do you think your service or you (as a staff member) would accommodate your own preferences if you were using the service? Is it even relevant to your service? How difficult would it be to accommodate your needs and preferences?

How well do you accommodate the needs and preferences of people with protected characteristics? Have you ever asked anyone whether you meet their specific needs or what could be improved? How far do you think services should go in meeting the needs of those with protected characteristics; what is reasonable adaptation?

What small changes could you (or your service) make to better meet the needs of people with protected characteristics? It can be something environmental, an activity, staff knowledge – let your imagine fly.

To get you started, would you know how to have a Rabbi visit and do people have to request this or would you offer? If you have ramps and wide doors in your scanning service, how do you ensure people can transfer to the couch? How do you adapt working arrangements for Muslim staff during Ramadan? Could you offer information in Braille?

Would you offer Halal meat? Do you celebrate Hanukah or Eid? What music do you play in your service? How do you manage where people prefer care to be provided by someone of the same sex? Do you ask?

_____

_____

_____

_____

_____

How well do you understand the usual practices of various religions or cultural groups? Do you stereotype people into categories that behave or want things a certain way? Would you know how to store the Qur'an in a respectful way? Do you assume there are no gay Catholics? Would you expect all Catholics to want to speak with a visiting priest? What would your expectations of a service user from the traveller community be? Where is your understanding from?

_____

_____

_____

_____

_____

From the Commission guidance for providers

How are people's privacy and dignity respected and promoted?

How does the service and staff make sure that people's privacy and dignity needs are understood and always respected, including during physical or intimate care and examinations?

Do staff respond in a compassionate, timely and appropriate way when people experience physical pain, discomfort or emotional distress?

I have lost count of how many exposed body parts I have seen, with and without the person's permission, over the years I have worked in regulation. There is very rarely a need for regulators to see body parts which are usually covered, but sometimes people seem to lose their inhibitions in certain settings, or with certain conditions, and sometimes staff have been thoughtless. I think the only time I have felt it necessary to see body parts that are usually covered was when an elderly person had been severely scalded and no appropriate treatment had been given. I described it earlier so won't go into detail. I needed to understand the severity of the wound to determine the level of expertise needed to advise on the care and treatment. That was more about my professional and moral responsibilities as a nurse and I was acting outside of the remit of a regulator.

Occasionally, inspection teams see people who are distressed and who want to talk to them but generally it is not within the remit to attend to those in distress and the best way to protect their dignity is by walking away, after ensuring staff are dealing with the situation. Slightly different where staff or service users want to talk to the inspection team but are distressed, of course.

Thinking about yourself, where is your comfort level around exposure of your body? It's a deeply personal thing and sometimes people are surprising when they reveal (sorry) their own inhibition level. It's maybe interesting to think whether nakedness compromises dignity or whether it is the lack of consideration and control which does.

How happy are you to be naked? What if it was somewhere fairly quiet and the only people around worked there? What about skinny-dipping somewhere isolated and beautiful? Bathing in front of your children, yes or no? Do you sleep or wander around the house without clothes or quickly swap day clothes for pyjamas in the privacy of your own room?

My story of being caught skinny dipping in the Newlands Valley by a large group of ramblers has entertained many others over time; we thought it hugely funny, but I know others who would have stayed in the water until everything went blue or fell off rather than walk past a crowd of about 30 people sitting close by to eat their cheese sandwiches and apples. In my defence we were young, so it wasn't too traumatic for the ramblers. We are all different; it's one of the joys of being human. If you have any inhibitions or discomfort about your own nakedness, why is that and how does it make you feel? Are there times you have felt particularly uncomfortable about it? Maybe with a new partner, with colleagues at a spa weekend, in communal changing rooms? How did you react?

How might you feel if you had nakedness or exposure forced upon you? If you had little choice because there was a requirement to be undressed in front of others? What might make it feel more tolerable? Does it matter if the person appears to not realise or isn't sufficiently cognisant to complain? Does it matter if it's only in front of professional staff?

Now think about your service and what you or your colleagues do to protect people's dignity.

Are there times where people's dignity could be compromised through being exposed beyond their comfort level? It might be wider than being undressed; it might be hair loss exposure, it might be shared accommodation or facilities, it might be visitors walking around. It could be waiting areas or being moved around the service or where there is a risk someone might have a seizure on trips out. It might be a lavatory opening straight onto a waiting area or having to sit around in a hospital gown for five hours before surgery.

It could be fathers staying overnight on postnatal wards leaving some women feeling uncomfortable. How do you manage that?

Where are the risks in your service?

_____

_____

_____

_____

_____

What do you do well to protect people from undue exposure or discomfort? Do you consider the different comfort levels that people have? How do you know how people feel? How can you evidence what you do well? At the other extreme, do you allow people to sleep without clothes, if they choose to so do?

_____

_____

_____

_____

_____

Now close your eyes and do a virtual walk of the journey that people take in your service – or think about a person's day in your service, if they are with you for some time. Imagine you are that person using the service.

What might make you feel uncomfortable, exposed or embarrassed? If in your imagination you are a bit embarrassed, how could this discomfort be addressed? What could be improved? It might be something to do with the building like moving a lavatory door away from the reception or it might be bigger gowns and wraps. It might be staff behaviours and routine. It might be better blinds in an ultrasound suite or moving intimate examinations from the patients' bed with just a curtain to a more private consulting room on a ward.

Don't think whether it is possible in reality – think whether something could simply be better.

What are the barriers to making improvements and offering people greater protection of their dignity?

What are the solutions to overcoming the barriers?

Who do you use as chaperones and why? When do you use chaperones? Do you always offer a chaperone? How does the chaperone interact with the person using your service? Would you automatically offer a same sex professional for an intimate procedure or would someone have to ask?

In an operating theatre, how would you react if someone requested an entirely single sex theatre staff team for cultural reasons – or indeed for any other reason? What if someone refused a male midwife or a male nurse to do a cervical smear? How would you react?

What about in residential settings? Are chaperones used when a staff member of the opposite sex is providing intimate care? If not, why not? Is it because people aren't given a choice or because they are not really aware of who is touching them? In the same setting would a visiting GP be offered a chaperone when examining someone of the opposite sex?

If a young teenager presented and was required to undress for any reason, would you accept their parent as a chaperone? Would that make a difference whether it was the same sex parent or an opposite sex parent?

It is much easier to provide evidence that a service is exceptionally caring in some settings. Which services do you think they might be and why is it, perhaps more difficult in other settings? How can you show you care in a fairly fast-paced or focused pathway setting?

Are there types of service users who automatically bring out the caring side of staff? Conversely are there those who it is hard to be caring towards? What could you do to 'go the extra mile'? How can you ensure that those who are challenging to care for receive compassionate care?

Are you more considerate of fear or anxiety in a frail elderly person, a young pregnant woman or a middle-aged man in a suit? What about a drunk, a homeless person or a person who is violent? Why is that? How can you recognise when someone needs reassurance, if they don't fit with your stereotype of who might be frightened? If you identify that behaviours may be due to anxiety, does it change the way you behave towards the person?

What training or support do you have or does your organisation offer staff in recognising and managing unwanted behaviour that may be indicative of distress or fear? Have you ever been taught ways of de-escalating conflict or aggression? Are there things you can do that reduce the risk to you and your own anxiety levels so that your response to unwanted behaviours is calming? Is there a difference in managing behaviours that may be due to a disease process such as dementia as opposed to alcohol or drug induced behaviours?

How are people assured that information about them is treated confidentially, in a way that complies with the Data Protection Act and that staff support people to make and review choices about sharing their information?

Do you talk to your family or friends about work and people who use your service? Are there limits to what you do or don't share outside of work? Might you share what had happened but not their name, perhaps? What if someone told you they'd been to school with one of your parents or siblings, would you mention it to the person they knew? Does it make any difference what type of service you work in or why a person was there?

When you are having professional conversations, where do you hold them and who is involved? Do you restrict information sharing to staff who really need to know? Who attends multi-disciplinary meetings and are they privy to details of a person's condition and circumstances when they aren't directly involved in that person's care?

Where do you make telephone calls? Can anyone overhear people's details or are you careful to ensure the conversation remains private?

What about people speaking at reception? How is their privacy maintained? Do they need to describe the reasons they are there to the reception staff in front of a queue of other people? That might be fine in a dental practice but less so in a GP surgery where someone is worried about rectal bleeding or thrush.

Thoughts? Has anyone ever walked the service user's journey? Have you stood at your own reception and described something deeply personal or embarrassing? Have you sat in your waiting area and listened? Have you stood near the nurse's station and simply listened?

Part 5: Is it Responsive?

Responsiveness

In healthcare settings one of the key lines of enquiry is whether people can access care and treatment in a timely way. This is not really a feature of adult social care environments but still worthy of consideration in terms of planning to meet the needs of the local community and how accessible and timely your services are.

Maybe for a domiciliary care service it is about contingency planning to ensure people's visits go ahead regardless of snow or flooding. In services for people with learning disabilities and/or autism, perhaps it is not about how easily people can access the service but how easily people using the service can integrate and use community facilities. There is a move away from large, closed communities in grand old buildings with acres of grounds, and towards more domestic, smaller units that provide an experience that more closely mirrors the life that most people experience.

It is also about how well the provider plans the service to promote access which allows the continued support of family and friends. A hospital providing specialist care for long-term conditions that are complex may offer a picturesque setting in glorious parkland, but people needing ventilatory support aren't able to access those and it is probably more important for their families to be able to visit without difficulty.

Many will recall, with dismay and some embarrassment, society's treatment of some of our most vulnerable and the BBC Panorama programme in 2011 which exposed the abuse of people at Winterbourne View hospital. In response to the investigation and government reports, the Commission made changes and in 2017 issued a policy statement for new providers of services for people with learning disabilities and autism called *Registering the Right Support*. This was the CQC's policy on registration and variations to registration for providers supporting people with a learning disability and/or autism. It is worth a read for all who provide for people with learning disabilities and/or autism, as it sets out the expectations of what a good service looks like and the key considerations when new services apply to register. It would be equally useful when reflecting on your own service and thinking about how you could move an existing service towards meeting the criteria for new services.

For acute hospitals, issues like Referral to Treatment Times also feature in Responsiveness but are not going to be specifically addressed, they are beyond the control and remit of individual staff members and need careful strategic, cross-trust planning to achieve sustainable improvements. There is scope to use reflection as a tool to drive improvements, but this would need to be a bespoke piece of work with the teams involved.

Describe the setting for your service? Is it beautiful? Is it in a town centre or is it sited rurally? What is nice about it? What are it's best features?

_____

_____

_____

_____

_____

Think about how accessible it is by car and/or by public transport. How close is the service to frequent, reliable, seven day public transport (or five day, if you close at weekends)?

How wide is your catchment or how far do people using the service or relatives have to travel to get to you? How difficult is that journey? Are there 'nightmare' roads that are often jammed? Are there frequent train delays or is there a long walk from a bus stop (remembering that 'long' for an athlete is different to 'long' for an elderly relative)? What is parking like? Is it free or is it expensive and still results in a long, uphill walk? How many appointments run late or are missed because of parking or transport issues?

_____

_____

_____

_____

_____

What do you do to overcome some of those difficulties? What attempts do you make to reduce the stress and frustration of poor public transport or a lack of parking? Are there any measures you could take to improve the situation and the impact of a difficult journey? Think widely, it might not be in your gift to build a new multi-storey car park, but it might be possible to have a system that took some of the stress out of the delays and avoided missed appointments. How easy is it to call and have the time changed if you are running late? How clear on your website are parking difficulties? Do people who arrive looking frazzled get offered a cup of tea and reassurance, so they are in a better frame of mind to judge your service fairly? Could you offer a lift from the station if you are in the depths of the countryside?

What adaptations do you make to enable people easier access to appointments? What adaptations could you potentially make? Do you offer appointments for specific cohorts to allow easier access or have appointments at different times to suit different groups? Do you ever take the appointments to the people using the service, rather than them having to come to you? Might you offer access to several professionals at the same time? Could you work with other similar providers in the area to provide wider access to services for specific groups?

How well do you meet the needs of harder-to-reach groups or those who simply have very busy lives – travellers, homeless people, parents with young children needing to do a school run, the frail elderly, commuters? What about being able to make appointments? How easy is it if you don't have access to a computer, don't have good use of English, have a learning disability or are deaf? Maybe walk the booking and appointment journey in your mind and think about the barriers and what might present challenges.

_____

_____

_____

What could you or your service do to make accessing and attending appointments easier? Would you, for example, consider having staff who speak a language that is common in your area working at times when those who speak the language can access the service? Could you have an interpreter attend on certain days and make that known? Could you offer staff the opportunity to take services, such as immunisation programmes, into community settings such as children's centres, playgroups or older people's mornings at the local leisure centre? Let your imagination fly – what in a perfect world could you offer?

_____

_____

_____

_____

_____

If you don't offer appointments but work with people who may need to attend appointments at other services, how could you make it easier for those you work with? How could you engage and work with other service providers to make attendance at appointments easier? How much control do your service users have over their appointments with visiting professionals? How do you support them to attend hospital or audiology appointments? Do they get the same access to healthcare services as people living in the community and, if not, why not? How could you make the access to healthcare more equitable?

_____

_____

_____

_____

_____

In 2017, a survey about access to services by the homeless, published by Cymorth Cymru, the umbrella body for providers of homelessness, housing and support in Wales, showed that more than two-thirds of respondents had not had a hepatitis B or flu vaccination and half the eligible female respondents did not have cervical smears or breast examinations on a regular basis.

The Office for National Statistics shows that there is a more rapid decline of good health, by age, among people who were less proficient in English.

What puts people off or limits people using your service, do you think? What are the barriers to people attending? This might be about groups or individuals who are underrepresented in terms of access to the service when compared to the local population.

Can you think of possible solutions to the challenges that people face in accessing services? Are there any steps you could take towards the solutions?
How might you sell the possible solutions or steps towards improvements?

Meeting individual needs

A one-size-fits-all health and care system simply cannot meet the increasing complexity of people's needs and expectations. This is being addressed nationally through the introduction of the NHS long-term plan, but it also falls to individual providers and individual staff to develop their own ways of working to ensure that individual needs are considered. That consideration includes but goes beyond the need to make reasonable adaptations for people with protected characteristics.

Consideration of your own work practice and your service, to ensure equality of access and outcomes, should underpin all that you do. This key question goes beyond that and encourages improving outcomes and the quality of services through the personalisation of care and treatment.

From CQC Key Lines of Enquiry

For healthcare services, including primary medical services:

How do people receive personalised care that is responsive to their needs?

How does the service identify and meet the information and communication needs of people with a disability or sensory loss? How does it record, highlight and share this information with others when required, and gain people's consent to do so?

Are the facilities and premises appropriate for the services that are delivered?

From CQC Key Lines of Enquiry

For adult social care services:

How does the service make sure that a person's care plan fully reflects their physical, mental, emotional and social needs, including on the grounds of protected characteristics under the Equality Act? These should include their personal history, individual preferences, interests and aspirations, and should be understood by staff so people have as much choice and control as possible.

Where the service is responsible, how are people supported to follow their interests and take part in activities that are socially and culturally relevant and appropriate to them, including in the wider community, and where appropriate, have access to education and work opportunities?

In this section, above all others, I think a simple tool can be used to really good effect. It's called 'Walk the Journey' and involves putting yourself in someone else's position to understand how they might experience your service and the care or treatment you provide. I know many executive and non-executive leaders do walk about and talk to patients and staff within trusts and independent hospitals. I know many care home owners or regional and corporate staff visit and do likewise. That's good, of course, but it's a missed opportunity.

I suspect that, when a senior person arrives, staff put on their best 'polite face' and make fairly bland comments. Self-censorship is, in my experience, common for a variety of reasons. Talking to someone who is breezing through the home, department, ward or other setting is not likely to give an accurate picture of the experience of individuals over and above whether lunch was nice or whether the problem with the laundry had been sorted.

Walking the Journey can take executive visits to the next level, they can also offer an independent perspective, if someone external to the setting is used. If you invite someone with a protected characteristic or specific need to walk the journey with you, the information will be much richer. Walking the Journey can also offer individuals and teams of staff an opportunity to really consider and think about how people experience the service and what the barriers (or indeed opportunities) to excellence might be. The idea could not be easier; walk the journey in reality or mentally, having put yourself in the shoes of a person using the service. Consider the details, use all your senses and think about it as an individual with a particular need or preference. Repeat from another perspective. If people need to undress at some point, imagine yourself being undressed in that setting and think about privacy, nervousness that there is no lock or that the door opens directly into a waiting area. If you imagine it from the perspective of someone with autism, think about noise, personal space and general 'busyness'. Don't assume the adaptations already in place are working or effective.

What do you understand by 'personalised care'? Is there a difference between a need and a personal preference, in respect of how much services should adapt to provide for those needs or preferences? What about where a personal preference is at odds with an assessed need?

_____

_____

_____

_____

_____

I have an affinity for cold water, I grew up on the coast and the love of swimming in the sea has never left me – even in November. I am convinced it brings real benefits in terms of both physical and mental health. You only have to see my husband and I squealing and giggling like teenagers in the sea off the Isle of Wight to know it generates joy. An 84-year-old woman living close to me still swims in the sea daily, on her own, year-round. Others might feel it poses real risks and might try to discourage her by citing cold water shock, cold incapacitation, drowning, cramp, hypothermia, falls, and no end of ills that might befall her.

Given her relatively advanced age, when should she be stopped from doing what she loves? When does the perceived risk matter more than her freedom to make choices and accept the risk? What pressure should be brought to bear to 'normalise' her? If she were living in a residential setting, would you still facilitate her daily swims? How would you want to reduce the risk – or might you want her to continue knowing that, for her, there are real health benefits to staying active, talking to impressed dog walkers, and from the cold-water immersion itself?

Where does your 'risk versus adventure and choice barometer' sit? Does it differ dependent on whether it is you taking the risk, someone you love or a person who uses your service?

What about within your service? Are you happy for people to manage their own risks (assuming capacity) usually, but less happy within your service?

_____

_____

_____

_____

_____

How do you determine what someone's needs and preferences are? What about someone who had capacity but who, due to illness or accident, now has reduced capacity? Do you take the relatives word about a person's preferences as valid and just go with that around things like favourite food, sugar in their coffee and activities? Do you check it out with the person themselves?

_____

_____

_____

_____

_____

_____

How accessible is your service in terms of access and facilities? Have you ever asked anyone with specific access needs what could be improved? Have you ever walked or imagined their journey?

Imagine now that you are reliant on a wheelchair and cannot transfer independently from your chair but can drive and operate your electric wheelchair yourself. Think through the journey into the service from car parking to lavatories; from where specific services are in the building and whether there is level access to getting changed or moving to an examination or treatment couch. What are the barriers and challenges? Can people who are reliant on a wheelchair speak at reception, use the lift buttons, operate drinks machines or open doors independently? A ramp and wide doors are not sufficient to say you have 'disabled access'.

_____

_____

_____

_____

_____

_____

Are there any immediate and simple improvements that could be made in attitude, arrangement or the premises that might make it much easier for someone who needed to use a wheelchair?

Which technology could you perhaps use to enable better access and more personalised care? Coronavirus has provided significant opportunities to innovate the way services are delivered. Could you use some of that experience to improve access? How might this be received? How could you find out whether it was something people wanted? These can be simple ideas such as online appointments to telemedicine to reduce the need for attendance at services.

There is a significant disparity between how most people can access services and how well someone with a learning disability accesses and experiences them.

An NHS Digital report from 2017 showed that, on average, the life expectancy of women with a learning disability is 18 years shorter than for women in the general population; and the life expectancy of men with a learning disability is 14 years shorter than for men in the general population. There is much work going on nationally to improve outcomes and reduce the variability in care, not least the Learning from Deaths Review programme, which is funded by NHS England.

What adaptations and considerations are given to the health needs of people with a learning disability or autism? How easy is it for people with a learning disability to make appointments, access your service and participate in preventative healthcare programmes such as screening? How easy is it for them to understand what is happening in your service? How many adaptations do you make? Is it all down to a carer attending with them? What oversight is there of their physical health, vision, dental care and hearing? Do you use the same referral guidance as for the general population?

In an acute, elective setting in which you don't have many patients with a learning disability, how well do you think you meet the needs of the few? Are you actually able to meet their needs fully or should you perhaps acknowledge that their needs are too complex for the setting as it is?

In a social care setting for people with learning disabilities, how much consideration do you give to healthcare? Is it only if 'something goes wrong' or there are obvious physical signs of ill health?
Describe what you do well.

_____

_____

_____

_____

_____

_____

_____

Can you think of any ways your service might be able to improve how well it provides or supports good healthcare for people with learning disabilities? Should it be proactive or reactive?

_____

_____

_____

Have you had training in supporting or treating the healthcare needs of people with a learning disability? What training do you think might be useful? Is there anything that would concern you about caring for or treating a person with learning disabilities in your service? Do you involve specialist staff, or do you think it is the responsibility of all staff?

The charity Dementia UK tells us that:

> *"Dementia is a global concern, but it is most often seen in wealthier countries, where people are likely to live into very old age. In 2014 there were over 850,000 people living with dementia in the UK. Of these, approximately, 42,000 were people with young onset dementia, which affects people under the age of 65. As a person's age increases, so does the risk of them developing dementia. It is estimated that the number of people living with dementia in the UK by 2021 will rise to over one million."*

Huge numbers, and I am sure that there are very few of us whose lives have not been touched by dementia in some way.

From your experience and perception, how does dementia usually present in your service? Is it a single characteristic that make you understand someone may be living with dementia, whether diagnosed or not? What do you think a person with dementia looks like and how do they behave? Do you have a mental image of someone with dementia?

How do you think arriving at your service feels for someone with dementia? What might be frightening or distressing, what might be reassuring and calming?

What do you do well to meet the needs of people living with dementia? How do you adapt your care or the service you offer? Does the stage of dementia make a difference? What support is there for the person using the service?

Where do you get advice and expertise about the best way to care for and treat people living with dementia? How do you know whether the adaptations you make are effective? Do you use them because everyone else does or have you thought through what might work?

How could the way someone living with dementia perceives, reacts to or experiences your service be improved? Do you ever ask families or the person themself what they want? How far would you go towards meeting their wishes? Would you change the red lavatory seat for a bright yellow one if that was what a person had at home? Would you give them a bone china cup and saucer instead of a plastic mug, if that is what they preferred?

What restrictions do you place on people living with dementia (other conditions you perceive as reducing their ability to make decisions) in your service?

Are restrictions put in place to mitigate risk or to make management easier? Do you insist someone with early stage dementia has someone with them when attending appointments? How do you balance that against a safeguarding risk and potentially hidden abuse, if a person has no opportunity to speak for themselves? Conversely, do you allow a familiar person to remain and provide support? If so, what are the limitations around this? What if someone said they wanted a soak in a deep, hot bath rather than a lukewarm shower? How might you manage that?

What if they were distressed in your theatre recovery area? How could you manage that? There will be scenarios for most types of services. Think about where you set limits that aren't really necessary but just 'the way things are done'.

How do you record information and evidence about what I would term, 'everyday consideration of personal needs and preferences'?

When the inspection team, senior managers, people who might potentially use the service or their families visit, how do you show them the responsive and individualised nature of your work? Do you just say, "We have passports" or, "We talk to their families when they first arrive"?

That's nice but not enough to really showcase what you do: nice is fairly commonplace, hopefully most people working in health and social care are nice. It's too woolly to have much impact and it says nothing about how much you personalise care. It's all well and good to have a policy for meeting individual needs, a dementia strategy, passports even, but how do you show what actually happens in practice?

How do you share the wonderful work you are doing among your own staff group, among other teams, with commissioners, with inspection teams and with prospective service users?

_____

_____

_____

_____

_____

_____

_____

What else could you do to share good practice more widely and build a positive impression with people using your service and their families? Think outside the box – there are no wrong answers.

_____

_____

_____

_____

_____

_____

Complaints and comments

In the Commission document entitled *Complaints Matter* (2014), the foreword by Professor Sir Mike Richards, then Chief Inspector of Hospitals, said:

> *"[Complaints] matter for people using services, who deserve an explanation when things go wrong and want to know that steps have been taken to make it less likely to happen to anyone else.*
>
> *They matter for health and social care organisations, because every concern or complaint is an opportunity to improve. Complaints may signal a problem – the information can help save lives, and well-handled concerns will help improve the quality of care for other people.*
>
> *Complaints matter to CQC, because they tell us about the quality of care. They tell us about how responsive a provider is, how safe, effective, caring and well-led they are. We can use our powers as a regulator to shine a light on good and bad handling of complaints and encourage organisations to improve."*

Any organisation that is setting its sights on becoming rated 'Outstanding' needs to understand that complaints are not necessarily a bad thing. Just as incidents are an opportunity for learning and reducing risk, so complaints handled well within a culture that wants to acknowledge shortcomings and put things right, are a very good opportunity for organisational learning and reputation building. Most complaints that reach the Commission are where people feel the service they have used hasn't listened or responded; they have felt fobbed off. Many people simply want an apology.

Obviously, a series of complaints about similar things suggest a more systemic problem and it is how the provider responds that is important. Putting the organisational head in the sand, minimising the impact on people, deflecting or denying a problem or dismissing service users as unreasonable is the very best way to avoid an 'Outstanding' rating.

As Professor Sir Mike Richards was oft heard to say, "Outstanding does not mean perfect".

What do you understand a complaint to be? Is it only where it is formal or are the smaller 'niggles' complaints? At what level do you record complaints?

_____

_____

_____

_____

_____

_____

_____

With the Key Lines of Enquiry for Adult Social Care

How are people's concerns and complaints listened and responded to and used to improve the quality of care?

How well do people who use the service know how to make a complaint or raise concerns and how comfortable do they feel doing so in their own way? How well are people encouraged to do so, and how confident are they to speak up?

How easy and accessible is it for people to use the complaints process or raise a concern? To what extent are people treated compassionately and given the help and support they need to make a complaint?

From GP Inspection Framework

Concerns raised by people using services, those close to them, and staff working in services provide vital information that helps us to understand the quality of care.

From healthcare provider Key Lines of Enquiry

How are people's concerns and complaints listened and responded to and used to improve the quality of care?

If someone complains about something, how does it make you feel? It might be something that seems very small, like their coffee being too cold or the car park being full. If it's something you consider more major, how does it make you feel? That might be a complaint that the nurses were talking and laughing loudly 'all night' or that their mother was sent home three times after being told she had a virus but ended up very ill in hospital with pneumonia. Does the nature of the complaint make you feel differently? What if the complaint was about you?

Does it make any difference to how you feel or your response if a complaint is made by someone who you know raises concerns quite frequently? Do you ever dismiss complaints (or recurrent concerns) because they are from a particular person? What do you think the risks of doing this in your type of service might be?

I would heartily recommend reading the *Report of the Independent Inquiry into the Issues raised by Paterson* (2020), available on the gov.uk website. The section on complaints is a good place to start when reviewing your own attitude and processes around complaints. Paterson was trained as a general surgeon, initially specialising in vascular surgery, but was nonetheless appointed as a specialist breast surgeon working for an NHS Trust in 1998. Paterson also practised as a surgeon at several hospitals in the independent sector.

He was suspended from practice in 2011. In April 2017, Paterson was convicted of 17 counts of wounding with intent and three counts of unlawful wounding relating to nine women and one man, whom he had treated as private patients between 1997 and 2011. Paterson was sent to prison for 15 years. His jail sentence was felt to be too lenient and was increased by the Court of Appeal to 20 years in August 2017.

The Inquiry found that, "Of the patients who told us they raised concerns with the trust, the majority were unhappy with how concerns were handled and the outcome of the trust's action. Patients told us they found the complaints process difficult and not well signposted, and they were put off by the timescales involved when they were looking for closure."

The report says that many patients felt the trust was too defensive and that responses to complaints did not always address the issues raised. This led them to feel the issue was not being treated with the seriousness it deserved. There was a belief among some patients and relatives that complaining would adversely affect ongoing and future treatment.

The report says that patients from the independent hospital, who did not complain said they either did not have the energy to do so or felt they would not be heard.

Among the patients and relatives who raised concerns with the independent hospital, the majority did not feel these were handled well. The provider was described as unresponsive and dismissive of its responsibility for the care patients had received.

The prosecution was a while ago now and there has been a commitment to improvement from the services involved, but are we now good at listening and responding to complaints?

If a complaint was made about another member of staff or visiting healthcare professional who you had a good relationship with, who was kind and popular, how might it influence your reaction to the complaint? Might there be an unconscious bias? How could you avoid that?

Imagine you are someone who uses your service and want to make a complaint. Do a mental walk through the process and think about how accessible and easy to use it is. Where are the stumbling blocks or barriers that would make you just give up in frustration? (I would be surprised if there weren't any!)

Do you even know the process?

Think about information for people, language, the perceived impact on care or treatment, the power imbalance, the format in which complaints must be submitted, the timescales and number of steps.

What steps do you take to avoid small niggles becoming big complaints within your service? What early intervention do you use? Who is involved and have they had training in complaint resolution? Is mediation available? Who is responsible for addressing the small niggles? Is local resolution recorded?

Where is the independence in the management of complaints within your service? How could you demonstrate that the process was fair and impartial; that the odds aren't stacked against the person complaining? Is there any external involvement (someone not employed by the service or provider)?

How do you share learning from complaints (including small niggles)? Would other staff know if Mrs Jones had said her coffee was often cold by the time it was handed to her or that Mr Smith was unhappy his front door was not pulled shut enough to lock properly? What about if Ms Johnson had complained that she had been seen by the trainee GP four times over a three month period for persistent bloating, loss of appetite and frequency but felt dismissed and hadn't yet been referred for any tests? How well do you really share the learning?

If you work with people who may feel a stigma attached to using your service, what extra steps do you take to ensure that they can raise concerns or complain, if they want to? How do you make it easier to complain? Do people have to approach you, or do you check how things are, for example? Are these groups of people less likely to be listened to and their concerns less likely to be taken seriously, do you think?

This will apply to many types of service but particularly to mental health services, sexual health services, termination of pregnancy services and accident and emergency or ambulance services providing care to people with mental health difficulties.

How could you improve the way you and your service encourage and respond to complaints? What would make learning from complaints easier?

_____

_____

_____

_____

_____

_____

_____

_____

What monitoring and follow-up action is there in respect of any complaints made (particularly the smaller, less formal complaints)? What is the governance of complaints in your service? Who looks for trends – particularly around informal 'niggles'?

How would you (or your service) know if Mrs Newton and Mrs Cuthbert were also unhappy about cold coffee or that four other women had made repeat appointments for potentially serious issues and felt dismissed by the trainee? Would you know if three separate relatives had raised similar concerns that their usually sprightly elderly relatives seemed very sleepy and uncommunicative during recent visits?

_____

_____

_____

_____

_____

_____

_____

What evidence do you record about complaints management and learning from complaints? How is this shared so that individual staff are aware of the learning and can give examples, if asked? As an individual staff member, do you feel you have a responsibility to seek out this information? Would you know where to look?

Part 6:
Is it well-led?

Who is a leader?

"If your actions create a legacy that inspires others to dream more, learn more, do more and become more, then, you are an excellent leader."
Dolly Parton

"Leadership is the art of getting someone else to do something you want done because he wants to do it."
Dwight D Eisenhower

Those not in leadership positions might well think this section doesn't apply to them. They would be wrong, of course, because leadership is not about a title. Leading is about striving to become better than we are, and helping everything and everyone around us to become better, too.

Being a leader is a very different thing to having a management title. Hopefully, within your service the managers and executives are leaders, but that is not universally true.

You may have heard of the Peter Principle, which first appeared in a book by the same name. The authors, Dr. Laurence Peter and Raymond Hull, suggested that workers in a hierarchical structure get promoted to the level at which they are incompetent and stay at that level for the rest of their careers. Logically, this might mean that virtually all managers are incompetent; if they weren't incompetent, they wouldn't be where they are but would have continued to progress. There is plenty of evidence to support the Peter principle, but that doesn't mean your organisation, or you need to adhere to the principle. Organisations who adhere to the Peter Principle are not going to get very far along the road to excellence.

My working definition of leadership is something like this:

> *Leadership is how a person influences others to do well and to achieve, and how they direct the organisation in a way that sees everyone supporting and agreeing the view of where the team wants to be.*

Many people can be leaders within an organisation. The very best organisations recognise that bringing those who have the greatest ability to influence others on-side and working with the designated leaders, is in everyone's interest. Using people with leadership skills to drive specific projects or to bring about improvements in their area or practice or interest can pay dividends. You don't have to be a CEO to be a leader.

You will probably have heard of Rosa Parks, the seamstress who helped initiate the civil rights movement in the United States when she refused to give up her seat to a white man on an Alabama bus in 1955. The Montgomery Bus Boycott began the day Rosa was convicted of breaching the segregation laws. Led by a young Martin Luther King Jr, the boycott lasted more than a year and ended only when the U.S. Supreme Court ruled that bus segregation was unconstitutional. Rosa Parks had no MBA, no Diploma in Management Studies, she wasn't high up a corporate ladder and had no title, but with her belief in justice and her determination to uphold the rights of all citizens, she changed a nation.

Is there the leadership capacity and capability to deliver high-quality, sustainable care?

Do leaders have the skills, knowledge, experience and integrity that they need – both when they are appointed and on an ongoing basis?

Do leaders understand the challenges to quality and sustainability, and can they identify the actions needed to address them?

Are leaders visible and approachable?

What is the leadership in your part of the organisation like? Is it shared, with everyone taking on specific responsibilities? Is there clearly one person in charge? Is there debate and discussion about how things are done and are different views listened to? Is the leader a bit too soft, perhaps, and wanting to keep people happy at all costs? Are there too many leaders and a confusing matrix of decision-makers?

What attributes, values, characteristics and skills would you want in your perfect manager?

Are there any characteristics or deficits you think would make a manager very difficult to work with or which would undermine the respect you might have for them?

If there is a need for something to be changed because of a situation outside local control – perhaps a change to shift patterns imposed by a corporate provider, new training and qualification requirements, new clinical guidance or a new IT system – how would you want those changes to be introduced?

Should the manager act in favour of the corporate or commissioning requirement or be solidly alongside the staff? Why do you think as you do?

Is it easier if it just happens and everyone has to get on with it, or would a slower, step-by-step change be better?

_____
_____
_____
_____
_____
_____
_____

Which characteristics of a good manager or leader do you think you have? How have you decided that you have the characteristics that you think you possess?

_____
_____
_____
_____
_____

What are your personal barriers to being a good leader, in its widest sense?

_____
_____
_____
_____
_____

I'll work through my list of characteristics which I think make a leader stand out from others on the crowded leadership platform (in a good way). For each, think about whether this is true of you as a member of staff in your organisation and how you demonstrate it. We can all show different characteristics depending on the situation we are in, which is why I think you need to consider how you behave in your workplace. As I mentioned before, leadership is not just for those in management positions – we can all contribute and help our organisation, or part of the organisation, grow with a resultant improvement in outcomes and culture.

Positivity. I think great leaders are optimists who see the good in things and help individuals and teams build on their strengths. I don't mean gushing, sycophantic sugar coating, but recognition and celebration of good practice; spreading a 'can do' attitude and a commitment to being the best. Positivity does not mean ignoring shabby behaviour or shortcuts; it means helping everyone improve by sharing the learning where things are working well. Whingers rarely change the world – but that is not to say people shouldn't raise valid concerns in the right way (see next characteristic).

When and how do you demonstrate a positive attitude towards your organisation, your team, your work and those you care for or treat? Do you share good news regularly? Do you help others who are struggling?

Doing the Right Thing – Integrity. The very best leaders in any setting are those who can be trusted, who have a strong moral compass and who are prepared to put their heads above the parapet, when necessary. People are forgiving of many things, but a perceived dishonesty or cowardice resulting in 'hushing things up' is a sign of weakness, not strength. Sometimes it is uncomfortable, sometimes it is quite risky, sometimes it is lonely, but knowing what's right and standing firm on that is essential. I can think of quite a few examples such as Rosa Parks mentioned earlier, and Emmeline Pankhurst who tolerated appalling treatment because she clung tight to her belief in universal suffrage. Her dedication and leadership of the suffragette movement bore the fruit that was the Representation of the People Act 1918, which gave voting rights to women over 30 years of age.

When do you show integrity? Have you ever found 'doing the right thing' difficult? Have you ever had to work against a culture of 'just good enough', or worse? How do you feel if people lie to you? How do you feel if you are short-changed in a shop or bar?

Why is integrity so important? Is 'spin', 'stretching the truth' or 'gilding the lily' ever acceptable?

Communicating well. What does this mean to you? Which famous people do you consider to be great communicators? I suspect people will name many different people.

Some will like Boris Johnson's style, with repeated slogans and his carefully crafted but informal style of communication. His speech is littered with 'we', so that people feel included and part of the solution; he uses words that have a strong appeal to patriotism. He tends not to use many facts and repeats his slogans many times to ensure they are embedded in people's minds.

Others may think that Barack Obama is a better communicator; he has a reputation as a great public speaker. Obama is an expert at delivery. From the moment he steps onto a stage, he beams confidence. You can see him scanning the audience and seeming to maintain eye contact with everyone. In his election speech his language was positive and talked of a dream – which maybe resonated with an American audience. He talked of a brighter future for the many.

If you dislike politics, then Greta Thunberg may be someone who you feel has captivated the world with her speaking. She's certainly memorable, brave and passionate. Her opening statements are bold. In her speech to the United Nations she said, "This is all wrong. I shouldn't be up here. I should be back in school on the other side of the ocean. Yet you all come to us young people for hope. How dare you?"

It certainly got the attention of many across the globe. If you listen or read the whole speech, it isn't flowing, it isn't particularly well crafted, but my goodness, it comes from the heart and is spewed out with passion aplenty. Sometimes, it's not about the words but about the humanity of the people who speak them.

Communicating is more than public speaking, it is more than words. What do you think good communication looks like? Are you a good communicator or, rather, when are you a good communicator? Many of us feel uncomfortable speaking in a meeting or on a stage but are very good communicators on a one-to-one basis. We may have an innate ability to engage children or to hold difficult conversations with people we work with. Where do your communication skills sit?

Are there times or situations where you find it difficult to communicate well, where you feel really uncomfortable?

Communication is a two-way process. How good are you at listening and why do you listen? No idea where I read it, but there was something I saw that asked whether you listened in order to respond or whether you listened to understand? Which do you think is most useful in building good communication between two people?

Decisiveness. Someone needs to make decisions and sitting on the fence rarely gets anyone anywhere. Good leaders are willing to take the risks associated with decision making; they make these decisions and take risks knowing that if things don't work out, they'll need to hold themselves accountable. Leaders don't look to abdicate responsibility for their decisions. Sometimes that is small decisions – deciding it's OK to go ahead with a barbecue because 'it's only a shower' isn't a massively poor decision, if there are contingency plans in place in case the shower becomes a downpour. Sometimes it's much bigger decisions and there can be a significant impact, if made unwisely. A good leader is still courageous enough to make decisions.

Indecisive leaders, who want every decision to be made by consensus are not leading. Consulting is good, bringing people with you is good but decisions made by committee with an attempt to please everyone and who allow debate to continue may well end up with a piecemeal decision that satisfies no one.

How decisive are you? Do you always seek reassurance from a colleague before making decisions? Do you worry about your decisions upsetting people? How do you make decisions? What level of consultation or discussion do you prefer? Does it matter what the decision is and what the level of risk is?

Think about a real-life difficult decision you have made recently. What was the decision and what were the risks? Did you consult and if so, who did you consult? Why did you seek the opinion of others? Was there guidance to follow that helped you make the decision? Do you believe you made the decision wisely and if you could go back in time and faced the same decision again would you have handled it differently?

Vision and strategic direction

What do you want in life? Where do you want to end up in ten years' time? Personally and professionally.

_____

_____

_____

_____

_____

_____

Do you have a plan about how to get there? Is it vague or specific? 'Be richer' or 'complete specialist training, apply for promotion and invest my inheritance in a buy to let property'? What steps to achieving your ambitions have you agreed with yourself?

_____

_____

_____

_____

_____

_____

What are the advantages of having something to aim for and identifying steps to reaching the end point? Are you a 'go with the flow' and see where life takes me type person who thinks it's all down to luck and circumstance, or do you think we have control over our own destiny? Is the same true of organisations?

_____
_____
_____
_____
_____
_____

Do you know what the ambition for your organisation or team is? Do you think it's a good ambition/vision? Is it realistic or just words? What do you like about it? Were you involved in deciding the end point? Do you think it is possible for your service to be among the very best?

_____
_____
_____
_____
_____

Do you understand how the end point is going to be reached? Do you know what the measures of success are? What sort of steps are you and your team taking to reach the end point? Is it realistic or just words on a letter heading? Do you 'buy in' to the vision? What would help you 'buy in'?

_____
_____
_____
_____
_____

Behaviour and values

How do you like those close to you (friends, family, partner, children) to behave? Are there things that they could do that would make you very upset or cross? What do you think the six most important behaviours or characteristics are in a friend or partner?

_____

_____

_____

_____

_____

If someone close to you behaves in a way that falls outside of your expectations, how do you address it? Are you more tempted to let it slip or do you address it? Do you 'tell them off/point out their errors' or do you say how it made you feel?

_____

_____

_____

_____

_____

Think back to the last time someone made you cross. Why was that and how did you react? Were you calm? Did you look at why you were angry? Did you blame them? Did you seethe quietly and sulk in private?

_____

_____

_____

_____

Are the behaviours and values the same as you would expect from people you work with? Are there many differences between personal relationships and professional relationships? Is that about familiarity, professional boundaries, being a different person at work and in private?

Which six behaviours or characteristics do you think people using your service, or their relatives, would think were most important? This might be residents, patients, family members, visiting professionals. How well do you meet those expectations individually and as a team?

What behaviours would you like to see more evident in your team or organisation? Are there any situations where the behaviours that you like in others are more prevalent?

Do you know what behaviours your provider/service leaders expect? How is this communicated? Are they reasonable expectations? Is there a clear behaviour framework or value base that everyone knows and understands? If your organisation has explicit behavioural expectations or values, do people adhere to them? Does everyone?

If there are times when the behaviours that are shown by one or more staff are less than ideal, what do you think the main causes are? Are you ever guilty of being less than perfect? When and why? What are the triggers? What do you do if you recognise your behaviour has not been ideal?

Are you an optimist or a pessimist and why? What has influenced you that makes you see the good in things rather than the problems? Does fretting change the outcome?

What does a really good day at work look like to you? When do you go home smiling? What makes you wake up in the morning and have a tingle of pleasure at the idea of going to work? I really hope something does.

What stops every day being a good day? What changes the day from being a good day where you sing and smile to a day when you frown or cry? Are you responsible for good days? Can you help overcome the barriers to positivity? Can you change the way you respond to the bad bits?

What could be done to make more days, good days? Think outside the box and think widely.

What one change would mean you smiled more often? What influence could you have over that? How could you spread positivity? Should you spread happiness, is it anything to do with work? How could being more positive improve care for others? For clarity, I don't mean hiding from bad news or care shortfalls. I don't mean sycophancy. I mean the joy of knowing a job has been well done.

Culture

Much of what this book has explored has related to culture. Certainly, equality relates to culture and any organisation that does not truly consider people as equal and where staff aren't comfortable with difference is unlikely to have a very positive culture. Organisations that focus on profit rather than people are unlikely to deliver exceptional outcomes and are, ironically, less likely to see their profits soar.

What even is culture? I think of it as the personality of the organisation. It's often described as 'the way things are done in an organisation'. It is the way things are really done as opposed to what the glossy posters say. It's the respect, the positivity and warmth which staff communicate with. It's the sense of belonging and the shared core values.

Skills for Care say on their website that:

Our 'Good and Outstanding care' guide found that services with these ratings had a culture that's fair, inclusive and transparent. For example they:

- put people who need care and support at the heart of the service
- ensure managers and leaders are dedicated to delivering high-quality care and support and act upon feedback
- ensure managers and leaders are open, visible, approachable and empower others
- embed a person-centred culture of fairness, support and transparency
- ensure managers and leaders encourage and support a strong focus on inclusion, equality, diversity and human rights
- ensure the workplace culture meets the needs of people who need care and support, staff and other stakeholders
- ensure problems and concerns are always a priority and are committed to resolving them.

Considering each of the bullet points above, how well do you demonstrate that you or your team works in the ways described? Do you think some of the points are unnecessary? Do you think the leaders and website say one thing but that the people delivering care and support service think differently?

_____

_____

_____

_____

_____

The "culture of a service is the key to good outcomes". What are the advantages to having a positive culture for staff, for people using the service and for the provider?

_____

_____

_____

_____

_____

Who creates the culture? Is it driven from above or is everyone responsible? Does it just happen? Do one or two people dominate in a smaller service or at team level? How much influence on local or team level culture do middle managers or team leaders have?

_____

_____

_____

_____

_____

What can you do to improve the culture of the workplace? How can you add positivity and improve outcomes? What influence do you have personally?

_____

_____

_____

_____

_____

What was the last kind thing you did? Was it at work or at home? When did you do something for someone else that you didn't have to do? It can be something tiny or something huge. Cutting an elderly neighbour's grass or making a junior doctor a cup of tea; baking some biscuits for work or buying the Big Issue. If you have to do something, it's not kindness although you may do it in a kind way.
How did it make you feel? For how long? Why did you do it?

_____

_____

_____

_____

_____

Has anyone been kind to you at work recently? What did they do? Again, big or small actions. How did that make you feel? I mean something over the requirements of their job. Maybe someone offered to give you a lift home in the rain, someone offered to stay late to let you get away early knowing you were struggling to juggle childcare and work commitments, or someone brought you in a birthday cake?

_____

_____

_____

_____

_____

How does feedback work in your organisation or team? Who gives feedback? Is it usually top down, or does it work in both directions and sideways too? Is it generally critical or positive? Is it public? Is it reserved for formal supervision sessions?

_____

_____

_____

_____

_____

Think back to the last piece of positive feedback you received. How was it given? Was it specific or vague ('It was good to hear you talking to Molly about her earlier life, to draw out some of her memories', as opposed to 'you were nice')? Was it given at the time or some time afterwards? Who gave it to you and how did it make you feel?

_____

_____

_____

_____

_____

Think about the last piece of positive feedback you gave to someone. How did you give it? Was it specific or vague? Was it to someone junior, someone senior or a peer? How was it received? How did it make you feel?

_____

_____

_____

_____

_____

When was the last time you offered direct, unsolicited, positive, feedback to your line manager or someone else in a senior position? How did they react?

How is the work you do recognised? Is it an organisation wide reward system, is there a local or team reward system? How do people say thank you (for particularly good pieces of work you do as opposed to a 'Bye, thanks')? Do leaders send thank you cards or write personal emails that can be used in professional portfolios? How would you like your work to be recognised?

Do you give feedback to visiting professionals or staff from different departments? Do you get to know staff outside your immediate team as individuals? How do you do that? Is it only senior staff who can comment or everyone? In large organisations, do junior staff feedback to senior staff? Would a healthcare assistant be able to tell a consultant that they thought the way they calmed Mrs Bishop was really skilful?

Does your service or part of a service feel welcoming and inclusive to other professionals? Do people say hello or introduce themselves? Are some people ignored more frequently than others?

I've lost count of the number of times I've wandered around or stood waiting for someone to acknowledge my presence; I prefer to wait for the staff to make the first move as it gives time to observe, to listen and to consider the culture.

_____

_____

_____

_____

_____

How does your service or team ensure that consideration of equality underpins the culture, both towards service users and staff? Do you feel that it is a meritocracy where people are appointed or promoted based on their abilities? How does your organisation promote a fair culture for all? How representative of the workforce are senior leaders or the board? Are appointments ever about a certain 'look'?

Are rotas managed fairly and the harder jobs allocated fairly, or is there a perception of favouritism?

_____

_____

_____

_____

_____

Do you feel that protected characteristics among staff are given fair consideration by others? How does this work in practice? Do observant Muslim staff have earlier shifts or work nights during Ramadan, so they can eat Iftar as soon as the sun sets? Are observant Jewish staff offered the opportunity to reach home in time for Shabbat?

_____

How could you influence how fair your organisation is, how committed to equality? Is it something you feel is important in your service or is it not relevant?

Might you feel differently if your employer decided that everyone had to work on Christmas Day and Boxing Day, or that only married women with young families could have time off in July or August?

_____

What involvement do you have in how the organisation is run? Are you asked your opinion? Are you able to be involved in making decisions that affect your work life? What control do you feel you have over your working life? If you are part of a large organisation, how much say do you have in how the service is provided? Is it something you can influence in any way?

_____

Raising concerns

One of the critical reasons for building an open and trusting culture with a shared understanding of acceptable behaviours, is about building an environment where staff feel comfortable to raise concerns and confident that action will be taken when necessary.

Thinking about yourself, are you generally comfortable raising concerns in your private life? Do you complain in restaurants if your food is cold? Do you return a jumper that has shrunk in the wash, despite being washed in accordance with the instructions?

Think about the last time you raised a concern or complained. How did you feel beforehand? How did you approach raising the concern? Did you do it discreetly or shouting in anger? How was the complaint/concern received? Was the problem sorted out? At what point does making a comment become 'raising a concern'? Is saying to the cook that the chicken is a bit pink still raising a concern? Is telling the ward manager that the shower in Bay 7 is dripping raising a concern? What about telling the outpatient manager that a consultant was wearing a jacket and tie – or telling the consultant directly?

How about with something more personal? Have you ever raised concerns about the behaviour of someone else? Maybe inattentive hotel staff, a teacher at your child's school, or someone making a lot of noise late at night. How did that feel beforehand? Did you get your message across easily or did worrying about raising it make you less clear and angrier?

_____

_____

_____

_____

_____

_____

Do you generally 'mind your own business' or do you act if you see something that isn't right? Think about the following situations and what you might do. What affects your decision about whether to act?

- A group of three boys, aged about 12, kicking another boy who is on the ground in a local park.

- A woman in a town centre with a baby in a pram, shaking a screaming toddler while shouting, "If you don't shut up, I'll give you something to cry about".

- A neighbour hosting a large children's birthday party while in lockdown due to Coronavirus.

- Two older youths taunting a rough sleeper who is lying in a shop doorway.

- A friend driving home from a group meal out, when you know they have drunk at least one bottle of wine.

_____

_____

_____

_____

_____

_____

Think now about the potential risk if you decided in any of these scenarios that it wasn't your business. What could the worst outcomes be? If you found out that the worst outcome had happened, how might you feel?

_____

_____

_____

_____

_____

_____

Now move your thoughts to your work environment. How comfortable are you raising concerns at work? What was the last concern that you raised or reported? It might be something small, maybe that liquid food like custard is far too hot or that the stair carpet was loose on the fifth stair. How easy was it to report and was the matter fully resolved? Were you listened to? What might have happened had you not reported it?

_____

_____

_____

_____

_____

If you are a leader or manager, what do you do to make it easy for staff to share concerns? Do you seek out and ask about concerns by recognising facial expressions or body language that indicate someone is cross or upset? Do you rely on reporting via electronic systems rather than face-to-face discussion (it can be both – I make no suggestion that the correct incident process shouldn't be followed, but we know that not everything is reported formally). How do you encourage staff to share concerns?

_____

_____

_____

_____

_____

How comfortable would you feel raising concerns about another member of staff? Would it make any difference if it was someone senior? What if it was someone popular? Would you raise it with the person first or with your line manager? What does your policy say?

What is the threshold of concern you would tolerate? Do you think your organisation would respond? Would you find it easier to report a mistake, a resourcing problem or poor behaviour? Would you think that the leaders in your organisation might react differently in each case?

_____

_____

_____

_____

_____

_____

Do you generally 'mind your own business' or do you act if you see something that isn't right? Think about the following situations and what you might do. Do you feel responsible for other people's behaviour or systemic problems? They might not be directly applicable to your setting, but I am sure you can consider a similar situation occurring where you work.

- You notice that a care record was changed to show a fall that wasn't mentioned until their spouse mentioned bruises on their face.

- When you are stocktaking, you notice that the number of temazepam capsules in the stock bottle appears to be low, but the main register doesn't show any being used.

- You see a senior member of staff shouting at a more junior member of staff in the staff room.

- You see a member of staff recording a video of a distressed patient who is being violent on their phone. When asked, they tell you it is so they can show the manager how challenging this person can be.

- You are told by a shift leader to put someone in incontinence pads as there won't be time to keep taking them to the lavatory.

Think now about the potential risk if you decided it wasn't your business. What could the worst outcomes be? If you found out that the worst outcome had happened, how might you feel?

If you had a magic wand, what three changes would you introduce to make your working life better?

Part 7:
From reflection to action

Looking forwards

"Well done is better than well said."
Benjamin Franklin

"It is well to preach as I do, with my lips. But you can all preach with your feet and by your lives, and that is the most effective preaching."
Charles Spurgeon

Reflection is the tool that helps us develop self-awareness and to learn from what we and others have done. Building on what we have identified as good practice through reflection is the next step. We need to develop a personal reflection methodology and build that personal model into a team model that improves our working lives and the outcomes of those we care for and treat.

Finding barriers and reasons for not doing something is all too easy; growing ourselves and our teams is much harder. It should be fun, the intrinsic personal rewards should be obvious once embedded, and the improvements in outcomes should follow. That is not an automatic process, although just reflecting may sometimes be enough to drive changes by heightening awareness.

Imagine spending hours cooking a fabulous beef wellington, wrapped in chicken liver pate and mushrooms before being encased in golden puff pastry. When you bring it out to serve at the table, it is beautifully pink and tender inside. You'd thought about what to serve to impress.

Everything seemed perfect but your guests just ate some vegetables and moved the beef around their plates. Most of the wellington went in the dog. The guests left telling you they'd had a lovely evening, but you knew they hadn't liked the meal. You were upset and then cross. You had the same guests for another meal some weeks later. This time you decided to serve a wonderfully aromatic tagine. They once again left having eaten very little, while the dog gorged on organic, locally reared lamb.

How do you think you could have prevented the disappointment you felt? How could you ensure your friends went home feeling full and thinking you were a skilled and considerate host? That bit is easy. If you had reflected, you may have considered there might be something they didn't eat or that they might have specific dietary requirements. You could simply have asked them. They might have told you they were pescatarian. At that point, you would understand but it wouldn't have changed the outcome unless you actually did something differently, unless you change what you did. If you stuck rigidly to your planned menu knowing they were not meat eaters, then the situation would continue. If you swapped to a salmon en croute, there would not be much extra effort needed on your part and your guests might have greeted the meal with sighs of pleasure, rather than exchanged awkward glances with each other. The only unhappy one will be the dog.

The key message is that reflection helps us understand but doesn't actually change anything. That bit requires a commitment to changing thoughts and ideas into action.

It might be that your organisation has a well-developed formal Quality Improvement programme already. A Personal Reflection and Action Method (PRAM) will hopefully sit alongside the wider QI programme and support it by changing the ways individuals and teams work and the amount of 'buy in' they offer.

It's a very simple idea that you can't change everything at once as you end up with overload. Achieving excellence requires effort and commitment over a long period. Every member of staff has to accept part of the responsibility for achievement; they need to work together to sustain improvements. A man running a marathon takes an average 55,374 steps and changing a culture or changing individual behaviour is undoubtedly a marathon rather than a sprint.

There are more complex cycles of using reflection to bring about organisational change, but PRAM has just four steps – just as the name has a four-letter acronym. Short and simple.

PRAM Personal Reflection and Action Method

P Position

R Reflection

A Action

M Monitor

Position

The first step is to think about the current position.

Think about a problem or identify a strength you want to build on. That might be something that went well. It might be a difficult conversation that you turned around.

It might be a behaviour you have seen in others. It might be professional – a promotion you didn't get – or it might be personal – a challenge juggling all your commitments.

Reflection

Find space and time to reflect on the position. Go down every possible nook and cranny where solutions and barriers might be hiding. Weigh up the pros and cons of all options, think not only of actions but feelings that might be created through action or inaction. Imagine how others are feeling and how your behaviour might impact on them. Try and think positively, to look to benefits and improved outcomes.

Search with your heart as well as your head. Most people understand the difference between right and wrong. Try and think what is right, it makes all decisions far easier. I can't promise it will always get you where you think you want to go, but it will always feel good.

Action

The doing bit. Translating the answers and information from your reflection into behaviours. These can be tiny steps, a commitment to changing your own responses, a decision to learn something specific, an agreement among a team to introduce a new way of doing something. There can be more than one action from each reflection.

Monitor

This means going back to the beginning and looking again at the position to see whether you or your team have moved onwards and upwards. You can record it in all sorts of ways to show your improvement trajectory but that takes us into the world of jargon, which I try to avoid.

I will suggest a few ways a bit further on but the best and most effective way to monitor is through honest reflection on where you are now related to the starting point. That won't feel terribly comfortable for people who like hard data and 'proof'. Individuals and small teams will know well enough and can take pride in their own journeys.

Hopefully, the quantitative outcome data will begin to show improvements in all sorts of ways and will appease the number crunchers. Sadly, while you might be able to demonstrate a correlation, you are unlikely to be able to prove a causal link. More jargon… so we'll leave that there and say simply that people who have been honest in their personal reflection will know whether it has made a difference.

As a starting point, I would think each person, having got this far, should think of just one thing they could change that would make life better for them or for others. The two are usually linked, so it doesn't really matter which way you look at it. I'll give a completed example.

As a team you might want to consider one thing you'd like to improve and work together to achieve that.

Personal Reflection and Action Model	
Position	Think of what it is you want to change or improve. It's the story that you are reflecting on.
Reflection	Take time to think about the position, and include: ■ What you feel ■ What the others involved might be feeling ■ What you would like any change to look like ■ What may have triggered the position ■ How your reactions may have impacted on the position ■ What might have been done differently ■ What positives you might want to build on ■ Whether there are any obstacles ■ Whether you need any support or resources
Action	Consider what you personally can do to change the position, the interpersonal dynamics, the outcomes, negative feelings and to boost positivity. Not what you can't do but what you can do.
Monitor	After a reasonable length of time (dependent on scale of change and action) return to the original position and think whether anything has changed. Consider not only measurable outcomes but improvements in relationships or your own happiness.

It is, of course, cyclical and once the monitor stage is reached, you need to either sustain and move on to a different reflection or consider alternative actions to reach the point you wanted to reach in your initial reflection.

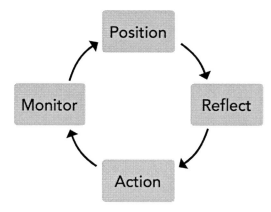

Personal Reflection and Action Model (Example 1)	
Position	I get cross when the cook is rude to other staff at supper time. She then sulks. It's always at the end of the day, when everyone is tired. She comes out and starts moaning at the nursing staff and telling them to hurry up so she can get washed up and go home. She's very impatient and clearly dislikes it when people want second helpings.
Reflection	I am probably tired at that point too. I have to stay late to ensure everything is settled and often have to meet with relatives after they have finished work. If I have to work late with a smile, I can't see why she can't.
	I suppose she does have to drop off and cook food for her elderly mother on her way home and maybe her mother worries if she doesn't arrive on time.
	She's not paid what I am either, so maybe she shouldn't have to work longer hours for free.
	It does take her a while to wash up and she is often late leaving. She does insist on everything in the kitchen and dining room being spotless before she goes.
	The other staff notice and talk about her all the time. She probably knows they don't like her. She certainly hears them telling people that she won't let them have second helpings.
	I've known it's a problem for a while and not really felt like tackling it. It ticks along OK and she is a very reliable staff member who cooks delicious food. That's sort of lost in her miserable personality though.
Action	I am the manager and it is down to me to help change the situation.
	Maybe I should talk to her about it – I will after the weekend and ask how I can make it better for her.
	It's not fair to expect her to work longer hours than she's paid for. Maybe we could change her hours to cover the lateness (although she still has to see her mother). I'll ask her when we speak if it might be helpful.
	Maybe it would be better to get someone in for a few hours a day to help with serving and washing up. I'm sure there are plenty of students from the college who would welcome three hours a day paid work. They'd learn the work then and could even cover if the cook were ever off sick.
	I wonder why she hasn't asked to take a hot meal from here to her mother. It would save her having to cook something separate and there is always plenty left over. Her mother is only around the corner and it would still be hot. It's very good food that she cooks.　　　　➔

Personal Reflection and Action Model (Example 1)	
Action (Continued)	Actually, I don't remember the last time I told her how good her food was. I must remember to thank her properly more often. I'll start next week when I talk to her.
	I think I'll mention in the staff meeting that we are going to have a new 'Star of the Week' staff member and the first one is the cook. I can remind them how reliable she is and how much people like her meals. I can mention how often she has stayed late to ensure all the jobs are done.
Monitor	Is it really three months?
	Cook is a different person. Seems she was not only cooking for her mother but paying for all the food as well. Letting her take a hot meal in a foil tray hasn't cost us anything but has apparently made a huge difference to her.
	People really like the 'Star of the Week'. We put their picture on the noticeboard and now relatives are telling me about particular staff members and what they have done. Its lovely.
	The assistant wasn't much use but cook says not having to rush to cook the meal and starting half hour later makes it manageable. I might persuade her to try another assistant, but I think I'd involve her in the recruitment process next time.
	The rest of the staff are nicer to her now I can just feel a difference when they are in the room together and instead of pointing out she won't let people have second helpings they point out what delicious food it is. She's even been getting to know the residents a bit better and is pouring drinks during the meal.

Personal Reflection and Action Model (Example 2)	
Position	It was really nice working with Matt, the new GP, last weekend. I went home laughing to myself. Usually, when I finish an Out-of-Hours shift I feel like a wrung-out dishcloth and can't sleep in case I have missed something.
	It was very busy, so that's not the reason, but we seemed to work more as a team. Maybe because he is new to OOH work, he checked in more about routines and wanting to check he was doing things properly. That meant I felt more comfortable checking out whether I was making the right decisions.
	Having our coffee together and allowing ourselves fifteen minutes without seeing patients gave us an opportunity to catch up. It was really →

Personal Reflection and Action Model (Example 2)	
Reflection	helpful as I could ask him about the child with a chest infection. I didn't worry I had missed a pneumonia.
	It's funny but I felt I knew him better than James who I have worked with lots of times. I think it makes it safer because we could both get a second opinion without feeling we were intruding or inept. Its reassuring sometimes.
	Maybe I was more open and friendlier towards him because he is younger, and I felt more on a level than with someone like James who is more experienced and older than me. I suppose James might not want to intrude on me or make me feel like he's questioning my judgments. Maybe he thinks we have nothing to chat about or thinks he can't offer to have coffee with me, in case its misinterpreted. Maybe if I asked for help, he might like sharing his knowledge; might be worth trying.
	I don't know if we have ever missed any potentially serious problems; we never really follow them up and don't really review how we are each managing patients. When we meet some of the team don't seem to engage much at all and don't seem to listen while others get really cross about the dishwasher and the milk. There doesn't seem to be real purpose to the team meetings, and they don't seem to help build relationships.
Action	I'm going to try and improve my relationship with the rest of the clinical team. I'm with Holly next weekend and James the weekend after.
	I'll start by offering them a coffee as I always get in half an hour before them. I can then suggest we take a coffee break together mid-morning and maybe talk about how I managed a couple of patients, to see if they would make the same decisions as me. They can only say no. They might think it's a good idea and we can then take it forward from there.
	If we have lunch together, I can ask how their morning has been and see if they need help with anything, I know Holly isn't always as comfortable as me in managing mental health problems.
	I can suggest we reserve part of the team meeting time for clinical review of specific patients to ensure that we do have an opportunity to share and learn from each other. It would be really good to know how James has managed complex situations and he might like presenting, to teach others. I'll email this afternoon and suggest it to others to see how they feel. Maybe we need a proper agenda.
	Not sure how we can follow-up and get a better idea of what our patient outcomes are like. Could we phone people or get feedback from GPs? Is there some way of checking whether they needed hospital later on? I think I'll ask at the team meeting. Others might know a way or have ideas.

Personal Reflection and Action Model (Example 2)	
Monitor	James is brilliant, he seems to know everything and has been really helpful. I feel so much more confident with him telling me I've done the right thing by the patients. Definitely worth making a few coffees for. I hadn't realised he was a gardener either and now I get regular gifts of fruit and vegetables. He says he much prefers feeling able to make suggestions, knowing I won't be offended. He even asked my advice about an infected leg ulcer last weekend.
	Team meetings are a bit better but it's still lots about unwashed mugs. We have agreed to have clinical supervision meetings once a quarter to present case studies and discuss management, which is a real step forward and maybe the clinical stuff wasn't so relevant to the admin staff.
	We still don't know what our outcomes are like, but the regional manager is going to discuss when she next meets with the CCG people. Maybe we could just get A and E attendance data for people who had been seen in OOH appointments within the preceding fortnight. Worth pursuing still.
	I wonder whether we should all sit in the handover at the end of each shift rather than just the lead GP? It would be a sort of debrief and ensure we had no loose ends.

It's really not difficult. It just requires an ability to think widely and recognise your feelings.

It can be done a bit more formally with a small team or group and an action plan with clear timescales and monitoring of the action plan, but for an individual you can simply use it as you choose. A written record is good for professional portfolio purposes and it is nice to look back and see what is achieved, it's almost like writing a diary and then updating on the diary entries but with a consciousness and intended actions rather than 'going with the flow'.

We choose how we behave and how we respond to any situation. That choice will impact on how others behave, and will affect outcomes.

What happens if you lack insight or can't consider others' perspectives easily?

It seems clear to me that the ability to look back with honesty and to consider all perspectives is key to using reflection to best effect. It's like self-coaching, and requires you to not only be the coachee but also the coach – if you are doing it individually.

If you cannot for whatever reason look objectively at a situation then you might need to consider alternative ways of making it work for you.

There are too many potential barriers to the successful use of self-reflection to list, some you may realise are a block, others you might not see as an issue. You might be too angry with someone to be able to consider how they are feeling. You might be too focused on what you want to achieve to see where the barriers or solutions to reaching that point lie. You might not like accepting responsibility for situations and be too ready to dismiss things as 'bad luck'. You might simply not be aware of factors affecting others involved in a given situation.

Finding a reflection partner, or someone to ask the questions that allow you to see the full circumstances and influencing factors of a situation more objectively, might help. Pair up and take turns to reflect. It can be about a shared experience (most useful) or completely different situations. What matters is that you listen to each other, don't offer solutions and don't say anything other than ask questions. Not, "Emily is finding her assignment really tough, you know, and is worried about not finishing on time" but more, "What do you think might have made Emily so impatient?"

I think the main way to improve your ability to use reflection is through practice. As with most skills, start with the simple things and gradually set yourself greater challenges. Personally, I'd start with things that went well. Maybe a really nice supper with friends; just before you are drifting off to sleep in a nice frame of mind, think back over the evening, the practicalities that worked, why it was such fun, what added to the pleasures and allowed the conversations to flow. Ask yourself questions and then answer them yourself. It really is that simple.

> *"Was the soup too spicy? It had a bit of heat, but everyone seemed to enjoy it, certainly the bowls were emptied. It nearly set my mouth on fire when I had the bread though. Maybe next time I won't do chilli bread as well. Actually, most people were full with the bread and soup – it was quite thick, so perhaps I won't do bread at all next time, just some croutons."*

Then when you have the habit of looking back and thinking about how you might do things a bit differently, you can move on to more challenging thoughts.

Reflective learning days/half days

These are always very well received in my own team, and there is much learning – although it isn't necessarily the learning that is planned as one never quite knows what will come up. The benefits are that the learning is entirely dependent on people's learning needs and as long as the culture and ethos of the days is set clearly, people can question or make suggestions without fear of getting something wrong or looking silly.

There is a training pack in the *Towards Outstanding* series that offers 'off the shelf' reflective practice day programmes and resources.

Choose your topic and plan the exercises

It needs to be relevant to your work and to your staff group. There is very little purpose in discussing antibiotic prescribing in an antenatal keepsake scanning service.

In many services it could be issues such as first impressions, safeguarding, dealing with complainants, managing verbal aggression, mental capacity and consent, promoting equality. The list is endless. Each service will also have specific areas of practice that could be used as the subject.

The exercises should be based on realistic practice or actual case studies. Clearly, they should be anonymous and in small services, it might be best to swop case study material with a neighbouring similar service. If two GP practices work together, then with a name change a person who failed repeatedly to follow advice might not necessarily be identifiable or use a historic case. In a corporate care home, it might be best for regional leaders or trainers to gather case studies from several homes and use those or staff from different locations.

Practically, you need to think of different ways for people to share best practice. So, a half day around medicines errors might be something like:

- **10:00 Icebreaker.** Nothing intimidating or designed to make people look silly.
- **10:30 Sharing in small groups.** 'When I made a medicine error'. Ask them to talk a little about the circumstances, how they realised, the impact and the

feelings they had when they realised. Encourage sharing about how they rectified the situation, whether they told the person concerned and learning from the event.

■ **11:00 Back together as a group.** Any common themes about when the incidents happened? Were people following their organisation's policy at the time? What do people perceive as medicines errors – prescribing errors? Omitted doses? Too long a course of treatment? Wrong timing of drug?

■ **11:30 Case studies.** Relevant to your setting. Three or four medicine error case studies with different outcomes and degrees of harm. Include issues such as hiding mistakes, accidental overdosage, missed dosage, incorrect calculation, maybe drug incompatibility picked up by pharmacist or missing controlled drugs. Ask groups to reflect on what the contributory factors might have been, how the staff might have felt, what the risks were, what the correct course of action would have been and what might be done to prevent a similar event happening again.

■ **12:30 Feedback** to whole group and wider discussion. One action to take away to improve practice.

■ **13:00 Lunch** or depart.

Find a facilitator. Not a tutor, not a leader, not an expert. Their role is to maintain a degree of structure around timings, to explain the exercises and to draw out discussions. It is often better to have a couple of people facilitating. Choose someone with a relaxed style.

If you are having several smaller groups for specific exercises, then ask people to chair those groups ahead, to avoid it becoming a hierarchy and to save time debating about who it will be.

Set the ground rules. You could spend half an hour agreeing them, but that is usually a bit stilted and artificial. I tend to just say them.
Ground rules are simple:

■ Non-hierarchical – everyone comes as equals and all views are valid regardless of their position in the organisation or professional expertise.

■ No question is too silly to ask. Experts may have an answer to a technical question but that doesn't mean they have the answer to everything.

■ Confidentiality must be respected (unless it is a safeguarding or misconduct issue).

■ Listen twice as much as you speak.

Deliver the day

Ask for feedback. Use to amend delivery of the next session. Offer attendance certificates for people's professional development files. Record on a training programme log to evidence staff training attendance.

Plan the next session...

Team time to reflect

This is a really easy mood booster and grows positivity in the simplest way possible. Team meetings are so often poorly led and can simply be a litany of things preached by a leader or manager – changes to policy, things not completed, Key Performance Indicator numbers, a moan about those dirty mugs or someone leaving a six-day-old tuna sandwich in the fridge. People walk away with their shoulders sloping, looking at the ground and feeling thoroughly miserable. Miserable staff are never going to deliver the best care.

Instead, set aside a few minutes at the very end of each staff meeting, leaders meeting, board meeting... any meeting. Literally minutes, depending on the size of the team. People should draw a numbered square of card from a hat (or a numbered counter from a teapot) and then, in chronological order, each person simply says one specific thing that has gone well in the past week or month. This should be something that has made them smile, something they are proud of, something they know they have done well.

It can start off a little awkwardly, but soon people are all smiling and saying how lovely something is or, "Wow, well done". Some will say, "That's a really good idea". Some will begin to feel pride in their work. Some will see the impact and pleasure that their good work brings to others. It's cheesy, perhaps, but it does help grow a positive culture that celebrates good news and builds on strengths. Everyone likes to be told 'well done', and there are few better ways to encourage staff to recognise the good work others are doing.

Personal pledge

It is what it says it is. At the end of the journal or at the end of a section of the journal, make a personal pledge to show how reflection has taught you something. Just one thing. It needn't be huge to make a difference. As Leo Tolstoy said, "Everyone thinks of changing the world, but no one thinks of changing himself".

Having reflected, choose just one thing you want to change about yourself. It shouldn't be something impossible to achieve or too self-deprecating. It should be one small commitment to make your life or the life of others nicer (the two are so often entwined).

If you're reflecting on first impressions, perhaps it might simply be to look visitors in the eye and say, "Hello, good to see you". It might be to take responsibility for the entrance hall noticeboard or to promise yourself to say, "Hello my name is" when meeting someone.

It might be to offer the junior doctor a coffee each morning. It might be to say thank you to each member of the team using their name at the end of each shift.

If you are working as a group, is a good idea to share the pledge. After a fortnight, check in to see how you are doing. Hopefully at the end of a month it will be embedded, and people will be able to see or feel a difference. Lots of small acts of kindness and good practice are far better at growing a positive culture than one huge magnanimous act that stands alone in a sea of grumpiness, ill temper, or harsh judgements.

As a team, or as an individual, you can log it or even display it proudly.

First Impressions Pledges			
Name	Pledge	two week reflection	One month reflection
Elspeth	To make sure the waiting area is kept tidy.	Thrown away any magazines over six months old or that were too tatty. Refreshed notice boards. Really enjoyed it.	Four people have said the waiting room looks better. The new children's toy box is popular. I like finding things of interest for the boards.
Pierre	Not to stockpile dirty mugs in my room.	I do clear them but several at a time. Jane told me off for just putting them in the staff room sink.	I found myself putting the dishwasher on for the second day in a row. Jane thanked me. A patient said my room looked cleaner.
Clive	To look up from my computer and make eye contact when listening to people.	Trying but more work to do. I just forget. Have a sticker that says 'Look up' now.	I find my consultations are going much better and I am looking at non-verbal clues more now. Its good to see people smiling sometimes. It feels more relaxed.

"Knowing yourself is the beginning of all wisdom"
Aristotle

Other titles in the Towards Outstanding series

For more information, visit www.pavpub.com

Towards Outstanding
A Guide to Excellence in Health and Social Care

The first title of this series, this is an essential guide for health and social care services that are regulated by the Care Quality Commission. Written by a senior CQC inspector, it shows how a mindset of getting the basics right then applying context-specific finishing touches can allow any service to drive improvement and move towards an 'Outstanding' rating. The author also explores why, in addition to other patient and organisational benefits, good care is cheaper to provide than poor care. Structuring her advice around the 'five questions' that CQC inspectors use (are services safe, effective, caring, responsive and well-led?), she draws on personal vignettes to paint a picture of a service where trust, positivity, a shared vision and a commitment to continuous improvement allow staff to generate new ideas, reflect on best practice, raise concerns where necessary and keep the patient at the centre of all activity.

ISBN: 9781913414696

Towards Outstanding
A Staff Training Resource for Health and Social Care

This resource is designed to facilitate and support the delivery of training for care services staff. Like other Towards Outstanding titles, it is built on the premise that reflection is a critical tool for driving improvement. Along with the core text *Towards Outstanding: A Guide to Excellence in Health and Social Care* (to which trainees require personal or shared access) and *Towards Outstanding: A Self-Development Reflection Workbook* (of which they should own a personal copy), it explains why reflection, assessment and continuous improvement are critical ingredients of exceptional care. With this foundation in place, a series of sessions spanning a wide range of topics allow staff to explore and collaborative plan the best way for their own organisation and team to move forward. Interactive and engaging, the wisdom and practical guidance contained in this resource can set any service on the road to an 'Outstanding' rating.

ISBN: 9781913414771

Towards Outstanding
Enabling Excellence in Care Home Provision

Outstanding residential care is personalised not packaged, and prevention is far better than dealing with the results of poor care. Yet driving improvement in service provision requires a process of continuous organisational learning to embed best practice. This unique resource provides all that is needed to create a framework for assessing a care home's strengths and weaknesses and taking the first steps on the road towards an 'Outstanding' rating. Drawing on decades of inspection experience, Terri Salt provides a suite of forms and templates that – with appropriate planning, discussion and collaboration – can serve as the basis for a full quality assessment as well as being built into a regular cycle of monitoring and continuous improvement. Using these tools, staff can learn to enjoy the experience of delivering the very best care to patients – and leaders can provide them with the tools and freedom required to do so.

ISBN: 9781913414818